The Hippocampal Region of
the Domestic Pig

Ida Elisabeth Holm

THE HIPPOCAMPAL REGION OF THE DOMESTIC PIG

A histochemical, immunocytochemical, and
morphometrical study

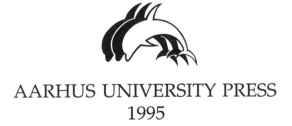

AARHUS UNIVERSITY PRESS
1995

AARHUS UNIVERSITY PRESS
University of Aarhus
DK-8000 Aarhus C
Fax (+ 45) 8619 8433

73 Lime Walk
Headington, Oxford OX3 7AD
Fax (+ 44) 865 750 079

Box 511
Oakville, Conn. 06779
Fax (+ 1) 203 945 9468

ANSI/NISO
Z39.48-1992

Denne afhandling er, i forbindelse med syv tidligere publicerede afhandlinger,
af det Sundhedsvidenskabelige Fakultet ved Aarhus Universitet antaget til forsvar
for den medicinske doktorgrad.

Aarhus Universitet, den 5. december 1994
Arvid B. Maunsbach
dekan

Forsvaret finder sted den 28. april 1995 kl. 13.00 prc.
i auditorium 424, bygning 230, Anatomisk Institut, Aarhus Universitet.

PREFACE

The present thesis is based on the following publications which are referred to in the text by Roman numerals:

I.   Holm IE, Geneser FA. Histochemical demonstration of zinc in the hippocampal region of the domestic pig. I. Entorhinal area, parasubiculum, and presubiculum. J Comp Neurol 1989; 287:145-163.

II.   Holm IE, Geneser FA. Histochemical demonstration of zinc in the hippocampal region of the domestic pig. II. Subiculum and hippocampus. J Comp Neurol 1991; 305:71-82.

III.   Holm IE, Geneser FA. Histochemical demonstration of zinc in the hippocampal region of the domestic pig. III. The dentate area. J Comp Neurol 1991; 308:409-417.

IV.   Holm IE, Geneser FA, Zimmer J. Somatostatin- and neuropeptide Y-like immunoreactivity in the dentate area, hippocampus, and subiculum of the domestic pig. J Comp Neurol 1992; 322:390-408.

V.   Holm IE, Geneser FA, Zimmer J. Cholecystokinin-, enkephalin-, and substance P-like immunoreactivity in the dentate area, hippocampus, and subiculum of the domestic pig. J Comp Neurol 1993; 331:310-325.

VI.   Holm IE, Geneser FA, Zimmer J, Baimbridge KG. Immuno-cytochemical demonstration of the calcium-binding proteins calbindin-D 28k and parvalbumin in the subiculum, hippocampus and dentate area of the domestic pig. Prog Brain Res 1990; 83:85-97.

VII.   Holm IE, West MJ. The hippocampus of the domestic pig: A stereological study of the subdivisional volumes and neuron number. Hippocampus 1994; 4:115-126.

ACKNOWLEDGEMENTS

The present studies were carried out at the Department of Neurobiology, Institute of Anatomy, University of Aarhus, Denmark.

I would like to thank first and most Finn Geneser for introducing me to the hippocampal region and for his never failing encouragement and enthusiasm throughout our collaboration. I am also very grateful to my other collaborators, Jens Zimmer and Mark West, for many hours of inspiring discussions. Special thanks are due to Dorete Jensen and Marianne Sørensen for technical assistance, Albert Meier for photographical assistance, Thorkild Nielsen for practical help with the animals, and Karin Wiedemann for secretarial help.

The studies were supported by the Danish Medical Research Council, grants nos. 12-8818 and 12-9740.

Ida E. Holm

Department of Neurobiology
Institute of Anatomy
University of Aarhus
DK-8000 Aarhus C, Denmark

CONTENTS

'The gains in brain are mainly in the stain'
Floyd Bloom

1. INTRODUCTION

The hippocampal region is a representative of the phylogenetically oldest part of the cerebral cortex, the allocortex. Since the classical Golgi studies of *Ramón y Cajal* (1893) and *Lorente de Nó* (1933, 1934) a large literature has emerged describing hippocampal morphology in many species. The hippocampus is clearly laminated into axonal, perikaryal, and dendritic layers and represents the least complicated type of cortex. For this reason, the hippocampus has proven ideal for studies of fundamental neurobiological problems, such as synaptic plasticity and neuronal excitability.

It is widely accepted that the hippocampus plays a prominent role in memory function (*Milner* 1970; *Squire* 1987, 1992). Its importance is exemplified by the profound amnesia found in patients following bilateral hippocampal injury after surgery, herpes simplex encephalitis or anoxia (*Scoville and Milner* 1957; *Victor et al.* 1961; *Volpe and Petito* 1985; *Damasio et al.* 1985; *Zola-Morgan et al.* 1986). Although the precise mechanism by which the hippocampus exerts its influence on the formation of memory is far from clear, it is believed that the hippocampus participates in storage of memory for variable time after learning (short-term memory) and enables consolidation of memory in other cortical regions (long-term memory) (*Squire and Zola-Morgan* 1991; *Eichenbaum et al.* 1992).

Various clinical conditions result in morphological changes in the human hippocampus. Of these, Alzheimer's disease, temporal lobe epilepsy, and ischaemia give rise to the most clear-cut pathological findings, whereas the hippocampus is affected to a lesser degree in schizophrenia (*Bogerts et al.* 1985; *Falkai and Bogerts* 1986; *Jakob and Beckmann* 1986) and Creutzfeldt-Jacob disease (*Misuzawa et al.* 1987). Alzheimer's disease is associated with the following pathological changes in the hippocampus: neuronal cell loss, neurofibrillary tangles, neuritic plaques, granulovacuolar degeneration, and Hirano bodies (*Katzman* 1986; *Tomlinson* 1992). The neuronal cell loss is most pronounced in the CA1 field, subiculum, and in layers II and IV of the entorhinal cortex (*Hyman et al.* 1984; *Arnold et al.* 1991) and corresponds with the highest density of neurofibrillary tangles within neurons in the region (*Hyman et al.* 1984, 1990; *Arnold et al.* 1991). Neuritic plaques are most numerous in the CA1 field, subiculum, and in layer III of the entorhinal cortex, but are also present in considerable numbers in the dentate molecular layer (*Hyman et al.* 1990; *Arnold et al.* 1991). It has been suggested that, as the disease develops and the pathological findings progress the hippocampus becomes functionally disconnected from its major afferent and efferent interactions (*Hyman et al.* 1984; *van Hoesen and Hyman* 1990; *Arnold et al.* 1991). Given the important role of the hippocampus in memory function, it is likely that at least part of the memory impairment observed in Alzheimer's disease is attributable to hippocampal damage. In temporal lobe epilepsy, the pathological findings in the hippocampus include a loss of neurons which is most severe in the CA1 field but also observed in the dentate hilus, the CA3 field, and the subiculum (*Sommer* 1880; *Dam* 1982; *Babb et al.* 1984). This cell loss may be very pronounced in patients with chronic epilepsy, then causing shrinking of the hippocampus termed hippocampal sclerosis. In addition, a loss of specific inhibitory neuron populations has been reported (*Babb et al.* 1989; *de Lanerolle et al.* 1989; *Sloviter* 1991) as well as synaptic rearrangements in the dentate area (*Sutula et al.* 1989; *Houser et al.* 1990). The sequence of events leading to the initial establishment of a seizure-inducing focus in the hippocampus is not clear, however, damage following febrile convulsions in early childhood is often mentioned as a possibility (*Meldrum and Bruton* 1992). The prevailing hypothesis explaining the loss of neurons in epilepsy is the excitotoxic hypothesis (*Olney* 1983), according to which excitatory neurons using excitatory amino acids such as glutamate as transmitter substance may destroy the cells with which they normally communicate, provided the excitatory activity is sufficiently intense and has a sufficient duration. It has been suggested that initial seizure episodes are particularly damaging to a class of inhibitory hippocampal neurons causing loss of inhibition which then initiates a cascade of destabilizing events ultimately leading to the loss of neurons and synaptic rearrangements (*Sloviter* 1991). With widespread loss of neurons, it may be easier to synchronize a large number of neurons, a key aspect in the generation of seizures (*Lothman et al.* 1991). Finally, the hippocampus is a classical predilection site for hypoxic-ischaemic injury in that the region is more susceptible to neuronal damage than other regions of the brain following short periods of global hypoxia or ischaemia (*Graham* 1992). The most vulnerable of the subfields are the CA1 subfield and the dentate hilus, followed by the CA2 field, the CA3 field, and, finally, the dentate gyrus (*Schmidt-Kastner and Freund* 1991). In addition, specific populations of inhibitory neurons are differentially affected (*Johansen et al.* 1987; *Johansen and O'Hare* 1989). Various hypotheses have been raised to explain the very complex cellular processes leading to hypoxic-ischaemic neuronal damage, i.e. the lactacidosis hypothesis, the calcium overload hypothesis, the excitotoxic hypothesis, and the oxygen-free radical hypothesis. Of these, the calcium overload hypothesis provides the best explanation of the mechanism of cerebral hypoxic-ischaemic damage although some of the other hypothetical mechanisms may play a secondary role (*Schurr and Rigor* 1992).

Most of the knowledge about the pathogenesis of the above mentioned diseases affecting the hippocampus has been gained through experimental pathophysiological studies using animals (e.g. *Price et al.* 1991; *Lothman et al.* 1991; *Schmidt-Kastner and Freund* 1991). The vast majority of these studies have been carried out in laboratory rodents and non-human primates. Those involving the former, primarily rats, have had the advantage of being able to draw upon the extensive body of descriptive and experimental literature that has emerged over the past decades. As animal models for human pathophysiological and toxicological phenomena, however, they are limited by fundamental differences between humans and rodents with regard to ontogeny and size and specific differences with regard to the internal organization of the hippocampal components. Although non-human primate models eliminate many of the problems related to species differences, they are encumbered by significant economical and ethical considerations that have limited their use. The hippocampus of the domestic pig (*Sus scrofa domesticus*) represents an alternative animal model for studying human disorders that has a number of advantages over the rodent and non-human primate models.

Domestic pigs have been used extensively in biomedical research because of the anatomical and physiological resemblance of a number of different organ systems to those of humans (*Douglas* 1972; *Dodds* 1982; *Tumbleson* 1986). They possess a relatively large, gyrencephalic brain which facilitates surgical intervention, the production of lesions, the installation of electrodes, and the placement of injections. As will be shown in this study, the hippocampus of the pig is in many ways more similar, than that of rats, to the hippocampus of humans. Although the hippocampus of non-human primates is structurally and perhaps functionally more closely related to that of humans and certainly the animal of choice for behavioural studies, the domestic pig offers many of the advantages of laboratory animals for experimental studies while providing a hippocampus that is structurally more similar to that of humans. Genetically, domestic pigs are as homogeneous as inbred laboratory rodents with the consequence that inter-individual variations are relatively small and experimental studies require fewer animals. In addition, the relatively large body size, which more closely approximates that of humans, makes it possible to more readily simulate human toxicological doses in these animals than in laboratory rodents or non-human primates. Perhaps more important for some laboratories, the ethical and economical considerations that accompany the use of domestic pigs are more similar to those involving the use of laboratory rodents than those involving non-human primates.

So far, the domestic pig has been the subject in several neuroanatomical studies (*Solnitzki* 1938; *Woolsey et al.* 1946; *Stephan* 1951; *Breazile* 1967; *Hereć* 1967; *Kruska* 1970; *Palmieri et al.* 1987; *Freeman et al.* 1988; *Niwa et al.* 1988; *Huffaker et al.* 1989; *Seeger* 1990; *van Eerdenburg et al.* 1990, 1992; *Østergaard et al.* 1992). With the exception of a few reports mentioning the hippocampal region of the domestic pig in other contexts (*Schaffer* 1892; *Dilberović et al.* 1986; *Kar et al.* 1989; *Palacios and Mengod* 1989), no comprehensive description of this region of the pig brain seems to be available.

1.1 Aims of the study

The aims of the study were therefore a) to make a comparative study of the hippocampal region of the domestic pig (*Sus scrofa domesticus*) with reference to other mammalian species previously studied, and b) to provide a description of the normal hippocampal region of the pig brain for comparison with data obtained from future experimental pathophysiological studies using this species as experimental animal.

The study includes a description of:
A. Architectonically and histochemically defined hippocampal subdivisions (I, II, and III).
B. The distribution of neuropeptide-containing nerve cells and terminals (IV and V).
C. The distribution of calcium-binding proteins (VI),
   and an estimation of:
D. The size of the hippocampal subdivisions and the number of neurons in these subdivisions (VII).

2. MATERIALS AND METHODS

2.1 Materials

The brains of young domestic pigs (Danish Landrace) (*Sus scrofa domesticus*) of either sex and with a bodyweight ranging approximately from 20 to 40 kg (8-14 weeks old) were used in the present study. We have chosen to use young pigs for merely practical reasons. In the domestic pig, puberty lasts from the 16th to the 30th postnatal week, and the pigs used in the present study therefore represent prepubertal pigs. Although the pig brain increases in size from 75% to 90% of the adult pig brain size between the 8th and 14th postnatal weeks (*van Eerdenburg et al.* 1990), no variation was observed in either the cytoarchitecture, the Timm staining pattern, or in the distribution of neuropeptides or calcium-binding proteins in the present study.

2.2 Methods
2.2.1 Histochemical Demonstration of Zinc (I, II, and III)

The Timm method (*Timm* 1958) is a histochemical technique that visualizes heavy metals, in particular zinc, which is primarily located in synaptic vesicles (*Haug* 1967; *Ibata and Otsuka* 1969; *Friedman and Price* 1984; *Pérez-Clausell and Danscher* 1985). The present modification of the method, the Neo-Timm method (*Danscher* 1981),[1] results in a more contrasted staining pattern with less nonspecific background staining than the original version (*Timm* 1958) and the more commonly used version by *Haug* (1973).

The method is based on the formation of silver deposits around zinc-sulphide complexes in the tissue. The density of silver grains shows a high degree of regional variability and the light microscopic appearance of stained tissue therefore varies between a yellow colour in areas with relatively few silver grains and a brown-to-black colour in areas with an abundant number of silver grains which then tend to coalesce. In the hippocampus, a particularly laminar staining pattern is obtained which outlines numerous interareal and interlaminar borders in the neuropil that escape detection in

---

1. For practical reasons, this modification is now referred to as the Timm-Danscher method, whereas the version by Haug (*Haug* 1973) is termed the Timm-Haug method and the original version Timm's method (*Geneser et al.* 1993).

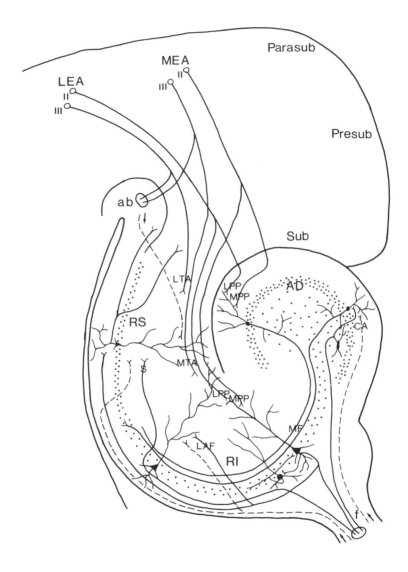

Figure 1. Schematic illustration of the major hippocampal afferent systems in the rat hippocampus. ab, angular bundle; AD, dentate area; CA, commissural-associational system; f, fimbria; LA, longitudinal-associational system; LEA, lateral entorhinal area; LPP, lateral perforant path; LTA, lateral temporo-ammonic tract; MEA, medial entorhinal area; MF, mossy fiber system; MPP, medial perforant path; MTA, medial temporo-ammonic tract; Parasub., parasubiculum; Presub., presubiculum; RI, hippocampal regio inferior; RS, hippocampal regio superior; S, Schaffer collaterals; Sub., subiculum; II, layer II entorhinal cells; III, layer III entorhinal cells. Full lines, ipsilateral connections; broken lines, commissural connections.

Nissl-stained material. This laminar staining pattern corresponds to terminal fields of known fiber systems (*Haug* 1975, 1984) and the Neo-Timm method therefore complements and very often extends classical morphological descriptions and definitions.

In brief, the animals were anaesthetized and perfused through the heart with a sulphide-containing solution. The brain was removed and the temporal lobes dissected and frozen with gaseous CO_2. 30 µm thick serial sections were cut in a cryostat and mounted on glass slides by thawing. The sections were prefixed in ethanol, rinsed in water, and then subjected to physical development. The developer consisted of filtered gum arabic solution, sodium citrate buffer, and hydroquinone dissolved in distilled water. Immediately before use, silver lactate in distilled water was added, and the solution was mixed thoroughly. The development was carried out in a dark box at 26°C for 60-70 minutes. After development, the slides were rinsed in water, postfixed in ethanol, dehydrated in ethanol, and finally cleared in xylene and coverslipped in Dammar resin. Counterstaining with toluidine blue was carried out in half of the Timm stained sections.

2.2.2   Immunocytochemistry (IV, V, and VI)

The main cell types in the dentate area and hippocampus proper include the dentate granule cells, the pyramidal cells of the hippocampal regio inferior and regio superior, and nongranule and nonpyramidal cells. The granule cells and pyramidal cells are organized in well defined layers, the granule cell layer and the pyramidal cell layer, and are the principal cell groups propagating activity in the hippocampus. The nongranule and nonpyramidal cells, on the other hand, are distributed in all hippocampal layers and are commonly regarded as the inhibitory element in the hippocampus (*Storm-Mathisen and Ottersen* 1984) since the majority of these cells contain the inhibitory neurotransmitter γ-aminobutyric acid (GABA) or its synthetizing enzyme glutamate dehydrogenase (GAD) (*Ribak et al.* 1978; *Storm-Mathisen et al.* 1983; *Somogyi et al.* 1984; *Gamrani et al.* 1986; *Sloviter and Nilaver* 1987) and form synaptic contacts on granule cells and pyramidal cells (*Somogyi et al.* 1983; *Kosaka et al.* 1984; *Frotscher et al.* 1984). The basic principles of hippocampal innervation are shown in Fig. 1.

In addition to the classical neurotransmitters such as acetylcholine, noradrenaline, dopamine, serotonin, histamine, GABA, glutamate, aspartate, and glycine, a number of small peptides with presumed neuromodulatory action (*Krieger* 1983) are also present in the hippocampus (*Storm-Mathisen and Ottersen* 1984; *Amaral and Campbell* 1986). Of these, somatostatin, neuropeptide Y, cholecystokinin, and vasoactive intestinal polypeptide are present in distinct subpopulations of nongranule and nonpyramidal cells and are therefore useful markers for different cell types (*Sloviter* 1989a), whereas enkephalin and substance P are primarily located in terminal fields. Furthermore, the calcium-binding proteins, calbindin-D 28k and parvalbumin, are also present in the hippocampus and can likewise be used as markers of cell types. In this study, the presence of somatostatin, neuropeptide Y, cholecystokinin, enkephalin, substance P, calbindin-D 28k, and parvalbumin was demonstrated using immunocytochemistry with the purposes of identification of various cell types, and formation of a basis for future experimental studies, since cells immunoreactive to these substances are differentially affected in pathological conditions involving the hippocampus. Furthermore, the staining patterns in the pig hippocampus were compared to those observed in other species, since it has been shown that the distribution of some neuropeptides is relatively well conserved throughout phylogeny (e.g. somatostatin and neuropeptide Y), whereas the distribution of others shows more clear interspecies variation (e.g. cholecystokinin, enkephalin, and substance P) (*Gall* 1990).

Immunocytochemistry was performed using the unlabelled peroxidase-antiperoxidase technique (*Sternberger* 1979). This technique is based on reaction of the antigen in the tissue with antiserum (primary antiserum) raised against the antigen. In order to visualize the antiserum-antigen complex a preformed enzyme-antienzyme immune complex (peroxidase-antiperoxidase) is linked to the antiserum-antigen complex in the tissue with a secondary antiserum added in surplus, and the substrate for the enzyme (peroxide) is finally added, together with a colouring agent. The peroxidase-antiperoxidase technique allows a qualitative identification of specific neuronal antigens which are visualized in direct topographical relation to the antigen-containing neurons. The technique is very sensitive and can be combined with other histochemical techniques. However, the visualization of any antigen depends on the specificity of both the primary antiserum and the immunocytochemical technique. Furthermore, to secure reaction of the primary antiserum with the antigen in the tissue, it is necessary to avoid that the fixation of tissue interferes with this reaction by destroying the epitopes on the antigen and insufficient penetration of the primary antiserum into the tissue (*Pickel* 1981). For these reasons it is necessary to conduct control experiments. These most commonly include specificity controls and staining controls. The specificity controls are performed by adding a surplus of antigen to the primary antiserum prior to incubation of the tissue containing the antigen. In case of specificity, no staining of the tissue should be seen. The staining controls are performed by omitting or replacing all of the antisera used, one at a time, as described below.

In brief, immunocytochemistry was performed as follows. The animals were perfused with fixative during anaesthesia. The brain was removed, postfixed, and a tissue block containing the hippocampal formation (including the dentate area, hippocampus proper, and the subiculum) along its entire septotemporal extent was dissected (IV, Fig. 1) and further divided into several smaller blocks from which 50 μm thick vibratome sections were cut perpendicular to the septotemporal axis. The sections were collected in several series scheduled for different staining procedures and were stored frozen in a cryoprotective fluid. Immunocytochemistry was then performed according to the unlabelled peroxidase-antiperoxidase technique. The sections were washed in buffer before a short incubation in serum. The sections were then incubated with the primary antiserum for 24 hours or 48 hours. After incubation, the sections were washed in buffer and then incubated with the secondary antiserum, washed again and incubated with a peroxidase-antiperoxidase complex. After further washing, the peroxidase was visualized with diaminobenzidine as a chromogen. After a final wash, the sections were mounted, dehydrated in alcohol, cleared in xylene, and coverslipped in Dammar resin. Half of the sections were in addition counterstained with toluidine blue. Control experiments included absorption controls for the visualization of somatostatin, neuropeptide Y, cholecystokinin, enkephalin, and substance P, whereas staining controls were performed for the visualization of all antigens. The absorption controls were conducted by incubation of the tissue sections with antiserum preadsorbed with antigen. The staining controls included omission of the primary antiserum, the secondary antiserum, the peroxidase-antiperoxidase complex, or all antisera, and replacement of the primary antiserum with nonimmune serum (*Larsson*, 1981). In addition to the absorption controls and staining controls, the presently used antisera were tested using the same staining protocol on sections from rat brains. The resulting staining patterns in the rat brains were identical with previous observations of the hippocampal region obtained in this and other laboratories.

Comparison of the distribution of immunoreactivity across species is often complicated by the use of different staining protocols in different laboratories. This includes variations in fixation of the tissue, use of different antisera that recognize different epitopes of the antigens, and variable use of colchicine pretreatment to enhance the staining intensity of nerve cell bodies. We abstained from the latter pretreatment in the pig for ethical reasons.

2.2.3 Morphometry (VII)

As a supplement to the qualitative description of the pig hippocampus, the volumes of the various subdivisions of the hippocampus as well as the number of neurons in these subdivisions were estimated using stereological techniques. Using the same technique, such studies have previously been performed in the hippocampal region of other animals, in order to make a quantitative assessment of changes in hippocampal size and neuron number during aging (*Coleman et al.* 1987; *West* 1993b) and in toxicological experiments (*Rungby et al.* 1987; *Slomianka et al.* 1989, 1992). In this study, the aims were to estimate the size of the hippocampal subdivisions and the number of neurons in these in normal pig hippocampi, and to compare these data with similar data from a variety of other species that vary significantly in size and degree of forebrain evolution (*West* 1990).

Recently developed stereological techniques (*Gundersen et al.* 1988; *West et al.* 1991; *West* 1993a; see also reviews by *Coggeshall* 1992 and *Mayhew* 1992) were used to obtain an unbiased estimate of the volumes of the hippocampal subdivisions and the number of neurons in these. In addition, the volume of the telencephalon was estimated, and the percentage of the telencephalon occupied by the hippocampus was determined.

Each brain was fixed by immersion into a mixture of glutaraldehyde and formaldehyde. The left hemisphere was embedded in agar and cut in 5 mm thick frontal slabs and was scheduled for estimation of the volume of the telencephalon. The right hemisphere was scheduled for estimation of the volumes of the hippocampal subdivisions and the number of neurons in these. The hippocampal region was removed from the right hemisphere, embedded in agar, and cut in 1.25 mm thick horizontal slabs. The slabs were dehydrated in ethanol and embedded in glycolmethacrylate. From each slab, one 40 μm thick section was then cut, mounted on a glass slide, and stained with a Giemsa stain before mounting using Eukitt.

The volumes of the telencephalon and the hippocampal subdivisions were obtained using the Cavalieri principle (*Gundersen et al.* 1988), according to which an unbiased estimate of the volume (V) of an object can be obtained from the sum of the areas of the individual profiles of the object on a set of parallel sections that are separated by a known constant distance (t). The areas of the profiles of the objects were estimated by placing a quadratic lattice directly over the object and counting the points at the intersections of the lattice (P_i) that hit the sectional profiles of the regions under consideration. The volumes were thus estimated as

$$V = t \cdot \frac{a}{p} \cdot \Sigma P_i$$

where a/p is the area of the grid associated with each point. The volume of the telencephalon was estimated using a transparent grid placed directly on the cut surface of the slabs of the left hemisphere, whereas the volumes of the hippocampal subdivisions were estimated using a grid placed on photomicrographs of the Giemsa stained sections.

The number of neurons in the hippocampus was estimated using a variant of the Optical Fractionator technique (*West et al.* 1991). This technique involved counting the number of neurons with optical disectors (*Gundersen* 1986; *West* 1993a) in a known fraction of the volume of each of the individual subdivisions. The optical disectors were systematically positioned in all three dimensions of each of the subdivisions so that all parts of the cell-body-containing layers of each subdivision had an equal probability of being sampled. The sections to be sampled were chosen in a systematic, random fashion along the dorsobasal axis of the hippocampus. This was accomplished by confining the sampling to sections taken from the corresponding surfaces of the 1.25 mm slabs that were cut from the hippocampus and ensuring that the placement of the first cut used to produce the slabs was random within the dorsalmost 1.25 mm of the hippocampus. Optical disectors were positioned in a systematic, random manner in each of the sections. This was accomplished by moving the slide under the objective of the microscope in a predetermined raster pattern with stepping motors attached to the stage of the microscope. The raster pattern comprised a number of x,y positions separated by predetermined distances along the x and y axes of the section. The first point in the raster pattern was randomly positioned within the first x,y interval to ensure a random placement of the raster pattern. At each x,y step, it was determined whether or not the counting frame superimposed on the field of view through a computer-video interface, was positioned over any of the neuron types to be counted. This was done by quickly focusing through the section. At positions where neuronal nuclei were seen under the frame, the plane of focus was moved 3 µm from the surface of the section into the section. The counting frame was then focused through 10 µm (h = 10 µm) of the section and the number of neuronal nuclei (Q^-) were counted using unbiased counting rules (*West et al.* 1991).

The area of the counting frame of the disector, a(frame), was known relative to the area associated with each x,y raster movement, a(x,y step). The latter was calculated from the size of the step movements made on the x and y axes ($\delta x \cdot \delta y$ = a(x,y step)). The areal sampling fraction (asf) was then a(frame)/ a(x,y step). The height (h) of the disector, that is, the excursion along the z or focal axis, was measured with a microcator mounted on the microscope. The fraction of the thickness of the 1250 µm thick slabs sampled by the disectors, the slab sampling fraction, was h/1250. The number of neurons in the subdivision (N) was estimated as

$$N = \Sigma Q^- \cdot \frac{1}{asf} \cdot \frac{1250}{h}$$

where ΣQ^- is the number of neurons actually counted in the disectors that fell within each of the respective subdivisions in the sampled sections.

3. RESULTS AND DISCUSSION

3.1   General Description and Terminology of the Pig Hippocampal Region (I, II, III, and VII)

3.1.1   Topology

The *hippocampal region* includes the *hippocampal formation* (*area dentata*, *hippocampus proper* (Ammon's horn), and *subiculum*) and the *retrohippocampal areas* (*presubiculum, parasubiculum,* and *area entorhinalis*). The retrohippocampal areas belong to the periarchicortex and are true multilayered cortices, whereas the constituents of the hippocampal formation belong to the archicortex and have a more simple structural organization. The hippocampal region occupies parts of the caudal and medial aspects of the hemisphere. The entorhinal area and part of the parasubiculum are visible with the brainstem and diencephalon in situ (I, Figs. 1-4), whereas the remaining parts of the region are only seen after removal of the diencephalon and brainstem (II, Fig. 1). The lateral border of the entorhinal area coincides with the rhinal fissure on the surface of the brain, and somewhat beneath the brain surface a medially directed additional fissure marks the true border between the entorhinal area and neocortex (I, Fig. 5, a). More basally and rostrally, the lateral border is against the prepiriform region. Dorsally, the rhinal fissure continues medially and slightly basally to reach the medial border of the hemisphere. The dorsal border of the entorhinal area and the parasubiculum therefore again is identical with the rhinal fissure in surface view, whereas the two areas abut neocortical tissue at depth. The adjacent presubiculum borders dorsally on retrosplenial cortex and ends more dorsally than the entorhinal area and the parasubiculum. Basally, the parasubiculum disappears before the presubiculum, which in turn ceases before the entorhinal area. The latter borders medially on the periamygdaloid cortex along the semiannular sulcus (amygdaloid fissure) and more laterally adjoins the prepiriform region. The medial edge of the retrohippocampal areas is represented by the rostral border of the presubiculum and lies on the medial aspect of the hemisphere a short distance from the hippocampal fissure (I, Fig. 5, d). On the medial surface of the hemisphere, only parts of the subiculum, dentate area, the hippocampal regio inferior, and fimbria are seen (II, Fig. 1), whereas the hippocampal regio superior is completely hidden due to the convoluted form of the hippocampal formation which is best appreciated on transverse sections (I, Fig. 5). The hippocampal formation forms a C-shaped structure along the medial aspect of the telencephalon curving dorsally and laterally to the thalamus. The

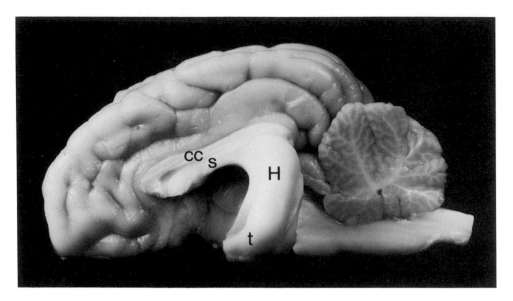

Figure 2. Left hippocampus of the domestic pig following removal of remaining part of the left brain half. cc, corpus callosum; H, hippocampus; s, septal part of hippocampus; t, temporal part of hippocampus. x2.14.

curved structure approaches the midline medially where it lies basal to the corpus callosum and caudal to the septum (Fig. 2). From here the hippocampal region curves laterally and slightly dorsocaudally for some distance, then bends and subsequently curves basomedially and slightly rostrally extending almost to reach the base of the brain caudal to the amygdala. The direction along the longitudinal axis of the hippocampal formation towards the septum is termed the septal end, whereas the opposite end is termed the temporal end. The subiculum does not extend as far septally as the hippocampus proper, which here bends medially to form the gyrus Andreae Retzii (IV, Fig. 1).

In other species, the position of the various components of the hippocampal region is basically identical with that described above in pigs. However, the extent of the hippocampal formation differs somewhat depending on the degree of encephalization. Thus, in rats the hippocampal formation is also C-shaped, but has a larger dorsal part which extends further rostrally and almost reaches the foramen of Monro just behind the septal area, whereas in primates, the entire hippocampal formation is located within the temporal lobe (*Rosene and van Hoesen* 1987). This shift from a C-shaped septotemporal extent in the rat to the temporal position in primates is caused by the greater development of the temporal lobe and the extension of the corpus callosum pushing the dorsal part of the hippocampal formation caudally in animals with progressive telencephalons (*Stephan and Manolescu* 1980). Thus, the position of the hippocampal formation in the gyrencephalic pig brain seems to indicate a degree of encephalization that lies between that of rodents and primates.

3.1.2 Cytoarchitectonics

The *dentate area* of the pig hippocampus (III, Fig. 1) is composed of the horseshoe-shaped *fascia dentata* and the *hilus fasciae dentatae* which is embraced by the fascia dentata. The fascia dentata includes the *molecular layer* and the *granule cell layer*. The following layers can be identified in the hilus: the *limiting subzone* [identical with the correspondingly named subzone of *Ramón y Cajal* (1893, 1968)], the *outer plexiform layer* [identical with the plexiform subzone of Ramón y Cajal], the *outer hilar cell layer* [identical with the second reflected blade of *Lorente de Nó* (1934) and with the subzone of fusiform cells of Ramón y Cajal], the *inner plexiform layer* [the cell-poor zone between the two hilar cell layers], and the *inner hilar cell layer* [identical with the first reflected blade of Lorente de Nó]. The terms medial and lateral are defined by the arrow (III, Fig. 1). At septal levels, the position of the two blades of the fascia dentata changes from medial and lateral to ventral and dorsal, respectively. The terms superficial and deep designate the directions towards the obliterated hippocampal fissure, and the direction towards the hippocampal regio inferior, respectively. The *hippocampus proper* of the pig hippocampus (II, Fig. 2) is divided into two major subfields, a *regio superior* and a *regio inferior*, in accordance with *Ramón y Cajal* (1893, 1968). Regio inferior is adjacent to the dentate area and is identical with the CA3 and CA2 regions of *Lorente de Nó* (1934) (CA: Cornu Ammonis, Ammon's horn), whereas regio superior is adjacent to the subiculum and corresponds to the CA1 region of Lorente de Nó. The layers within the hippocampus proper correspond with those described by *Ramón y Cajal* (1893, 1968), *Blackstad* (1956), and *Geneser* (1987a). These layers are not easily seen in Nissl-stained material but will nonetheless be mentioned here. The most superficial layer (i.e., the layer bordering on the obliterated hippocampal fissure) is *stratum moleculare*, followed by *stratum radiatum*, the *pyramidal cell layer*, *stratum oriens* and finally, the *alveus* which represents the deepest layer (i.e., adjacent to the surface of the lateral ventricle). In regio inferior, the *layer of mossy fibers* separates stratum radiatum from the pyramidal cell layer. The *subiculum* of the pig hippocampus (II, Fig. 2) consists of the *plexiform layer* and the *cell layer*, the deep part of which borders on the angular bundle or deep white matter. The *retrohippocampal areas* of the pig hippocampus (I, Fig. 5) all consist of six layered cortex. The layers are numbered consecutively I-VI from the surface of the brain. The *presubiculum* is located between the subiculum and the wedge-shaped *parasubiculum*. The *entorhinal area* is divided into two main parts, a medial termed *pars medialis* and a lateral termed *pars lateralis* according to the terminology of *Blackstad* (1956).

The most conspicuous comparative differences in the organization of the dentate area are found in the degree of lamination of the hilus fasciae dentatae. In the hilus of both the rat and mouse, no clear lamination is evident and the hilar neurons appear to be homogeneously dispersed. In contrast, in the guinea pig, rabbit, monkey, and humans, the hilar neurons are segregated in distinct laminae as seen in the pig dentate area (*Gall* 1990). The definition of the hilus has long been a subject of controversy. With the nomenclature used in the present study the outer hilar cell layer of the pig hilus corresponds to the more widely used "layer of polymorphic cells", whereas the inner hilar cell layer by some authors is termed CA4 cells, an incorrect use of the nomenclature defined by *Lorente de Nó* (1934), according to which CA4 corresponds to the outer hilar cell layer, the inner plexiform layer, and the inner hilar cell layer of the present study. Based on connectivity studies in the monkey, it has been shown that the two cell populations differ, in that the outer hilar cells (the polymorphic cells) give rise to the commissural-associational projection to the inner third of the dentate molecular layer, whereas the inner hilar cells (the CA4 cells) project out of the hippocampal formation to the septal area. For this reason, it can be argued that only the outer hilar cells (the polymorphic cells) belong to the hilus, while the inner hilar cells (the CA4 cells) should be regarded as modified pyramidal cells of the hippocampal regio inferior (for further discussion of this issue see *Rosene and van Hoesen* 1987). A determination of whether or not this is the case in pigs will have to await the results of similar connectivity studies in this species. We have included the inner hilar cell layer in the hilus in this study following the convention of *Geneser* (1987b). Comparative differences in the organization of hippocampus proper include variations in the degree of migration of pyramidal cells into stratum oriens and in the definition of the border between the hippocampal regio superior and the subiculum. In the pig hippocampus, a moderate migration of the deep pyramidal cells into stratum oriens in regio superior is seen, whereas the superficial pyramidal cells remain tightly packed, and the border between regio superior and the subiculum is rather well defined. In comparison, the pyramidal cells in the rat hippocampus show only little or no migratory displacement into stratum oriens in regio superior, and the boundary between regio superior and the subiculum is easily seen. Primates, on the other hand, show migration of the deep pyramidal cells into stratum oriens in both regio inferior and regio superior. This is most pronounced in regio superior, where the superficial pyramidal cells also appear loosely packed, and the border between regio superior and the subiculum is less easily defined (*Stephan and Manolescu* 1980; *Rosene and van Hoesen* 1987). Another comparative difference is seen in the hedgehog hippocampus, in which the layer of mossy fibers extends through both regio inferior and regio superior, particularly at temporal levels (*Gaarskjær et al.* 1982). The same phenomenon has been described in some strains of cats (*Laurberg and Zimmer* 1980). Comparative differences in the organization of the entorhinal area include a further subdivision of the two main parts in the guinea pig (*Geneser-Jensen et al.* 1974), rat (*Haug* 1976), and cat (*Krettek and Price* 1977), whereas the monkey entorhinal area is divided into seven main parts, primarily oriented along a caudorostral axis (*Amaral et al.* 1987).

3.2 Timm Staining Pattern (I, II, and III)

The characteristics of the Neo-Timm staining pattern in the pig hippocampal region vary somewhat depending on the level studied along the dorsobasal (septotemporal) extent of the region and are summarized in the following based on the appearance at middle dorsobasal levels.

In the *dentate area* (III, Fig. 5), the *molecular layer* can be divided into three sharply defined sublaminae corresponding to the outer (or superficial), intermediate, and inner (or deep) third of the layer. The outer sublamina appears stained with medium intensity, whereas the intermediate sublamina is extremely pale. The inner sublamina is stained with medium intensity in its outer part, but the intensity decreases gradually towards the granule cell layer to reach a weak intensity just superficial to the latter. In the *granule cell layer*, the superficial two thirds are well stained with a reticular appearance of the staining due to stained granules filling the interstices between the unstained cell bodies, whereas the deep third is almost unstained. Recurrent mossy fiber collaterals are often seen traversing the layer. The *hilus* generally appears intensely stained, although the various layers display extreme differences in the staining. The limiting subzone has the same staining character as the deep part of the granule cell layer and cannot be identified in either Neo-Timm or Nissl-stained sections. The outer plexiform layer is very narrow and can only be identified in some sections. Where present, the layer appears lightly stained with an admixture of coarse granules and fibers. The outer hilar cell layer is very intensely stained and appears almost homogeneously black. This staining most likely represents stained mossy fiber giant boutons in very large numbers causing confluence of the precipitate. Cell bodies, when distinguishable, appear unstained. The inner plexiform layer is weakly stained and is traversed by numerous darkly stained mossy fibers. The inner hilar cell layer is well stained with a reticular appearance caused by bundles of intensely stained mossy fibers converging towards the hippocampal layer of mossy fibers separated by lightly stained patches of different sizes. Cell bodies in this layer appear weakly stained.

In the *hippocampus proper, regio inferior* has the following characteristics (II, Fig. 4). *Stratum moleculare* is divided into a superficial, weakly to moderately stained sublayer and a deep, almost unstained sublayer. The superficial sublayer gradually becomes slightly more weakly stained towards regio superior and increases in staining intensity to medium towards the dentate area. The deep, very light sublayer is very narrow near regio superior, but widens towards the dentate area. *Stratum radiatum* generally stains weakly and contains vertically oriented, unstained strands which are particularly numerous in the superficial part of the layer. A narrow, almost unstained zone is present immediately superficial to the layer of mossy fibers. Nerve cell bodies appear moderately stained. The *layer of mossy fibers* stains very intensely and appears virtually homogeneously black along most of its longitudinal course. The initial portion, adjacent to the dentate hilus, appears looser in character, particularly in the infrapyramidal portion of the mossy fiber bundle which is present here. The main, suprapyramidal portion tapers near the transition to regio superior. The homogeneous black staining represents confluence of precipitate in a large number of intensely stained mossy fiber giant boutons, whereas individual, intensely stained mossy fiber giant boutons are only recognizable in the more loosely arranged portion of the layer. The *pyramidal cell layer* appears medium to darkly stained due to staining of the cell bodies, whereas the interstices between the cell bodies are relatively poorly stained. A few of the stained cell bodies are displaced into stratum oriens, where they appear randomly scattered. Near the dentate area, the layer attains a loose character and the increased space between the cell bodies is here seen to be occupied by stained mossy fiber boutons. Near regio superior, a decreasing staining reaction is seen of the cell bodies situated deep to the tapering portion of the mossy fiber bundle. *Stratum oriens* stains weakly with a slight decrease in intensity towards regio superior. Adjacent to the dentate area, the superficial part of the layer is occupied by the infrapyramidal portion of the mossy fiber bundle. In addition to the mentioned few, dislocated stained pyramidal cell bodies scattered at varying depths of the layer, smaller stained nerve cell bodies of an oblong shape are occasionally seen near the alveus, oriented parallel with the latter. The *alveus* appears very pale. In *regio superior, stratum moleculare* generally stains weakly, but a tapering process of darkly stained tissue projects from the plexiform layer of the subiculum into the deep part of stratum moleculare. *Stratum radiatum* in general shows a weak staining intensity, but has a superficial, lighter appearing zone which is most prominent adjacent to regio inferior and is characterized by vertically oriented unstained strands, separated by better stained neuropil. Immediately superficial to the pyramidal cell layer, a very narrow, almost unstained stripe is additionally present. Most of the very few nerve cell bodies present in stratum radiatum are moderately stained. The *pyramidal cell layer* appears as a medium stained narrow zone due to stained granules occupying the narrow interstices between the cell bodies which appear lightly stained. A substantial number of the cell bodies are displaced into stratum oriens. In *stratum oriens*, a very weakly stained, narrow infrapyramidal zone is present, and the remaining main part of the layer is subdivided into a superficial and deep subzone, each constituting roughly one half of the vertical extent of the layer. The superficial subzone stains weakly, whereas the deep subzone is intensely stained. The deep subzone tapers some distance from regio inferior and disappears immediately before reaching the latter, whereas it widens slightly in the vicinity of the subiculum. The superficial subzone is inhabited by unstained dislocated pyramidal cell bodies. However, the zone of dislocated cell bodies narrows gradually in the direction towards regio inferior.

The *subiculum* (II, Fig. 4) stains very well, but the staining pattern is more complex than the cytoarchitecture would seem to indicate. The *plexiform layer* has a weakly stained superficial subzone which comprises more than the superficial half of the layer adjacent to the presubiculum and is reduced to less than half of the vertical extent of the layer near regio superior. In addition, the subzone becomes more weakly stained near regio superior. The remaining deep subzone of the layer forms a considerably better stained subzone which is particularly dark near regio superior, whereas it exhibits medium staining intensity adjacent to the presubiculum. A narrow, almost unstained stripe separates the superficial and deep plexiform subzone, except near regio superior. The *cell layer* generally is well stained, and can be divided into three parts of roughly equal size along the presubiculohippocampal extent of the subiculum on the basis of differences in staining intensity of both the cell bodies and the neuropil. Near the presubiculum, the part abutting the deep layers of the latter stains with medium intensity with an admixture of evenly distributed, dark dots representing intensely stained subicular pyramidal cells. Towards regio superior, the part of the subicular cell layer adjoining the one just described shows intense staining reaction due to intense staining of both the subicular pyramidal cells and the intervening neuropil.

The remaining part of the cell layer near regio superior stains with medium intensity, although superficial and deep tongues of more intense staining are seen adjacent to the hippocampus. The nerve cell bodies appear almost unstained, whereas the neuropil generally is moderately stained, but in addition, darker stained vertical streaks are seen. In the superficial and deep, more heavily stained tongues adjacent to the hippocampus, the cell bodies remain unstained, whereas the neuropil shows more intense staining reaction. The deepest part of the cell layer towards the white matter is characterized by a wide transitional zone of weakly stained neuropil, in which scattered, well stained nerve cell bodies of an oblong shape are seen, oriented parallel with the white matter.

The *presubiculum* generally stains moderately and in a distinctly laminar manner (I, Fig. 9). *Layer I* stains weakly in its superficial half with the exception of the superficialmost part of the layer where a very narrow, more intensely reacting band is seen in the part of the presubiculum adjacent to the subiculum. The deep half of layer I stains with medium intensity. *Layer II* stains with medium intensity adjacent to the parasubiculum, where the staining of the deep half of the molecular layer continues without change in intensity into the interstices between the nerve cell bodies of layer II. The majority of these cell bodies exhibit moderate staining in this part of the presubiculum. Towards the subiculum, the staining of both the neuropil and the nerve cell bodies decreases and a narrow zone of pale character appears between the cell bodies and the dark inner half of layer I. In some sections, the nerve cell bodies of layer II tend to form groups, giving rise to darker islands consisting of better stained nerve cell bodies and neuropil separated by less intensely reacting neuropil. *Layer III* generally stains rather weakly, but has a somewhat inhomogeneous appearance due to the presence of apparently randomly distributed, darker staining small patches representing irregular areas of densely stained neuropil. Nerve cell bodies mostly appear weakly to moderately stained, but scattered, intensely reacting cell bodies are present in the small, dark patches. *Layer IV* forms a strongly reacting band, contrasting to the much lighter stained neighbouring layers III and V. The dark band is caused by intensely reacting neuropil and nerve cell bodies, but more moderately stained cell bodies are also present. *Layers V and VI* both stain weakly and cannot be recognized as separate layers.

The *parasubiculum* has a very characteristic appearance in that its outer part is seen as an intensely stained triangle wedged in between the entorhinal area and the presubiculum (I, Fig. 9). *Layer I* is divided into an outer, weakly stained half and an inner, very heavily reacting half, separated by a very narrow, virtually unstained stripe which forms a continuation of the one seen at the same laminar level in pars medialis of the entorhinal area. The inner, intensely stained half forms the outer portion of the dark parasubicular triangle. *Layers II* and *III* constitute the deeper part of the dark parasubicular triangle. *Layer IV* has a very short anteroposterior (mediolateral) extent and appears moderately stained. *Layers V* and *VI* cannot be defined, as these layers are seen to continue essentially unchanged from the entorhinal area into the presubiculum.

The *entorhinal area* generally stains very well, but with considerable differences in intensity from layer to layer and even within single layers, resulting in a characteristic laminar staining pattern (I, Fig. 9). In *pars medialis*, *layer I* stains weakly in its superficial half, whereas the deep half is medium to heavily stained. A very narrow, almost unstained zone is present at the transition between the superficial and deep halves, being most conspicuous in the medial half of the transverse extent of the layer. *Layer II* has a clearly lighter appearance than the deep half of layer I, due to the almost complete absence of staining of nerve cell bodies (stellate cells) and the lower density of stained particles in the neuropil occupying the interstices between the nerve cell bodies as compared to the inner half of layer I. *Layer III* shows medium to heavy staining intensity throughout the entire vertical extent of the layer, and most of the pyramidal cell bodies are moderately stained. *Layer IV* stains weakly and is identified as a light zone immediately deep to the much darker stained layer III. Most of the nerve cell bodies (horizontal cells) are weakly stained. *Layers V* and *VI* are weakly stained although slightly more so than layer IV, and it is not possible to distinguish the two layers as separate entities. Many medium or even heavily stained nerve cell bodies are, however, present. In *pars lateralis*, the staining pattern in many respects differs from that described for pars medialis. In *layer I*, the outer half remains unchanged except for disappearance of the narrow unstained stripe at the transition to the deep half. The latter is slightly less stained than in pars medialis. *Layer II* is essentially unchanged, whereas *layer III* is clearly lighter than in pars medialis. However, the deepest part of layer III remains well stained, although it appears a bit lighter than in pars medialis. *Layer IV* stains slightly darker than in pars medialis, the intensity being identical with that of *layers V* and *VI*, which remain unchanged. The darker staining of layer IV is to some extent caused by the presence of a greater number of well stained cell bodies than seen in pars medialis.

For comparison, the Timm staining pattern in the hippocampal region has been described in detail in several other mammalian species, including the rat (*Haug* 1974, 1976), guinea pig (*Geneser-Jensen et al.* 1974), European hedgehog (*West et al.* 1984), rabbit (*Geneser* 1993), monkey (*Macaca mulatta*) (*Rosene and van Hoesen* 1987), and humans (*Cassell and Brown* 1984). However, in the hedgehog, monkey and humans, no description of the retrohippocampal areas is available. Furthermore, the staining pattern in the human hippocampal region is of much lower quality than in animals because sulphide perfusion is impossible and formation of zinc-sulphide complexes in the tissue is achieved either by exposure of tissue sections to a sulphide solution (*Tauck and Nadler* 1985; *Chafetz* 1986) or gas (*Jaarsma and Korf* 1990), or by allowing postmortem autolysis during which endogenous sulphides accumulate in the tissue and form complexes with zinc (*Danscher and Zimmer* 1978). Either of these alternatives to sulphide perfusion results in a somewhat blurred staining pattern in which most often only the mossy fiber system (the dentate hilus and the layer of mossy fibers) can be identified with certainty. Comparison of the staining pattern in the pig hippocampus with that of the above mentioned species shows a fundamentally similar overall staining pattern, although closer scrutiny reveals clear interspecies differences. The differences include variation in staining intensity and sharpness of interareal or interlaminar borders in the neuropil and, apart from the variation in localization and density of the hilar mossy fiber boutons which is considered below, cannot be accounted for in structural terms. Rather, these differences reflect interspecies variation in the distribution and density of zinc-containing afferent terminals (boutons) in the hippocampus. Such differences in distribution and density of both commissural and associational connections have been reported to exist for the hippocampal region, even between species of the same order (*Hjorth-Simonsen* 1977; *Hjorth-Simonsen and Laurberg* 1977; *van Groen and Wyss* 1988). More extensive treatment of species differences in hippocampal connectivity is given by *Rosene and van Hoesen* (1987) and *Gall* (1990). An example of the differences is the variation seen in the dentate molecular layer which in all of the mentioned species, except monkeys and humans, appears trilaminar when stained with the Timm staining method. In rats, the outer third of the dentate molecular layer corresponds to the termination of the lateral perforant path (LPP) arising in pars lateralis of the ipsilateral entorhinal area, whereas the middle third corresponds to the termination of the medial perforant path (MPP) arising in pars medialis of the ipsilateral entorhinal area (*Hjorth-Simonsen* 1972; *Hjorth-Simonsen and Jeune* 1972; *Steward* 1976), and the inner third corresponds to the termination of the commissural-associational system (CA) arising in the ipsilateral and contralateral polymorphic hilar neurons (*Zimmer* 1971; *Hjorth-Simonsen and Laurberg* 1977; *Laurberg and Sørensen* 1981) (see also Fig. 1). In rats, guinea pigs, rabbits, and pigs the outer and inner thirds stain with medium intensity, whereas the middle third stains weakly, and the limits between the laminae are very distinct. In contrast, monkeys display a very sharply defined and densely stained inner third and weakly stained middle and outer thirds without clear distinction, whereas in hedgehogs, the outer and middle thirds appear stained with medium intensity while the inner third appears unstained. This lack of distinction between the outer and middle thirds in monkeys and hedgehogs might be a result of the different architecture of the entorhinal area and, hence, different distribution of connections. The dentate hilus in all species studied appears very intensely stained due to the large numbers of stained hilar mossy fiber boutons. There is, however, considerable species variation in the appearance of the staining pattern which in the pig, guinea pig, rabbit, monkey, and humans appears distinctly stratified with extreme differences in staining intensity between single layers, and in the rat and hedgehog appears homogeneous. In the species with stratified staining pattern, the stratification is identical and corresponds to the cytoarchitectural organization of the hilus which in these species is highly laminar, as mentioned previously. Conversely, the species with a homogeneously stained hilus show no lamination and the hilar neurons instead appear homogeneously dispersed. The difference in the Timm staining pattern of the hilus between pigs, guinea pigs, rabbits, monkeys, and humans on the one hand and rats and hedgehogs on the other therefore essentially displays the variation in the cytoarchitectural organization of the hilus and the concomitant variation in the distribution of the hilar mossy fiber boutons.

Until recently, the Timm method has been used almost exclusively for descriptive studies and in studies of either reorganization of the terminal fields of hippocampal afferents following lesions, or changes in terminal field sizes during phylogeny and development. However, two recently introduced techniques (*Howell and Frederickson* 1990; *Slomianka et al.* 1990) have enabled identification of the neurons that give rise to zinc-containing pathways, i.e. neurons that contain zinc in the synaptic vesicles of their boutons, and a detailed description of the distribution of zinc-containing neurons and their possible connections and terminal fields within the hippocampal region has already been performed in the rat (*Slomianka* 1992). The presence of zinc in synaptic vesicles (*Haug* 1967; *Ibata and Otsuka* 1969; *Friedman and Price* 1984; *Pérez-Clausell and Danscher* 1985) suggests that this metal may be involved in neurotransmission. This is supported by the findings that stimulation of hippocampal slices results in release of zinc (*Assaf and Chung* 1984; *Howell et al.* 1984; *Charton et al.* 1985; *Aniksztejn et al.* 1987), and ultrastructural evidence of a time-dependent displacement of zinc from synaptic vesicles to synaptic clefts (*Pérez-Clausell and Danscher* 1986). Several reports have associated zinc with glutamate (*Wolf and Schmidt* 1983; *Crawford* 1983; *Slevin and Kasarskis*

1985), opioid peptides (*Stengaard-Pedersen et al.* 1983; *McGinty et al.* 1984), and nerve growth factor (NGF) (*Crutcher and Davis* 1982; *Kesslak et al.* 1987), and more recently, interest in the physiological effects of zinc has focused on the interaction between zinc and glutamate-receptor types on the one hand and GABA-mediated responses on the other. In vitro studies have shown that zinc causes a depression of NMDA-receptor responses (*Peters et al.* 1987; *Westbrook and Mayer* 1987; *Forsythe et al.* 1988; *Koh and Choi* 1988; *Christine and Choi* 1990) and a potentiation of non-NMDA-receptor responses (*Peters et al.* 1987; *Koh and Choi* 1988). The distribution of zinc corresponds well with the anatomical localization of NMDA-, and non-NMDA glutamate receptors (*Cotman et al.* 1987), and zinc is without doubt co-localized with glutamate in the mossy fiber projection (*Bramham et al.* 1990; *Crawford and Connor* 1973) and probably also in the projection arising in the hippocampal pyramidal cells, and in the entorhinal lateral perforant path projection (*Slomianka* 1992). By virtue of the morphological and physiological relationship between zinc and NMDA-activated neurotransmission, zinc has been implicated as contributing to the induction of long-term potentiation (LTP) (*Weiss et al.* 1989), which is assumed to represent the electrophysiological basis for synaptic plasticity and memory storage mechanisms. Zinc also has been reported to cause inhibition of $GABA_A$-receptor responses (*Westbrook and Mayer* 1987; *Smart and Constanti* 1990; *Smart* 1992) as well as modulation of the binding of GABA to $GABA_B$-receptors (*Turgeon and Albin* 1992). However, there is no indication that zinc and GABA are co-localized in the hippocampus, as there is no overlap between the distribution of zinc and the localization of GABAergic neurons.

3.3 Neuropeptides (IV and V)

The neuropeptides somatostatin (SS), neuropeptide Y (NPY), cholecystokinin (CCK), enkephalin (ENK), and substance P (SP) were visualized using immunocytochemistry. The resulting staining includes immunoreactive nerve cell bodies and terminals. Immunoreactive cell bodies are characterized by a homogeneous or granular reaction product in the perinuclear cytoplasm and the most proximal parts of the neuronal processes. They have the structural characteristics of nongranule and nonpyramidal cells of the rodent hippocampus and are therefore classified according to *Ribak and Seress* (1983), *Amaral* (1978), and *Schlander and Frotscher* (1986). Immunoreactive terminals are present both as a distinct staining of fibers which are studded with varicosities and usually without direct relation to parent cell bodies, and as stained puncta of variable density. The number of stained cell bodies and terminals as well as their distribution in the hippocampal region vary considerably depending on the neuropeptide in question, and characteristic staining patterns are therefore obtained for each of the neuropeptides. Furthermore, the appearance of the staining pattern for each neuropeptide also varies depending on the level along the septotemporal axis. The following summary is based on the appearance at middle septotemporal levels.

Somatostatin-like immunoreactivity (SS). The SS staining pattern is characterized by a large number of intensely stained nerve cell bodies and faintly stained puncta and fibers. In the *dentate area*, a characteristic distribution of stained nerve cell bodies and terminals is seen (IV, Figs. 2b, 3b, 9). In the *molecular layer*, small cell bodies are occasionally seen in the outer two thirds of the layer. Puncta of low density and a loose plexus of fibers are also present in the outer third of the layer, whereas the deeper parts of the layer are occupied by fewer fibers. The *granule cell layer* is characterized by a few, small cell bodies embedded in the deep part of the layer, resembling pyramidal and horizontal basket cells, and scattered fibers crossing the layer. In the *hilus*, a large number of cell bodies is seen in the deep part of the outer hilar cell layer, the inner plexiform layer, and the superficial part of the inner hilar cell layer, resembling fusiform and stellate cells. A dense plexus of fibers is seen in the outer plexiform layer and outer hilar cell layer, whereas a less dense network of fibers is present in the inner plexiform layer and inner hilar cell layer.

In the *hippocampus proper* (IV, Figs. 2b, 3b, 13, 16), *stratum moleculare* is characterized by large, stellate cell bodies which are occasionally seen at the border towards stratum radiatum in regio superior. Puncta of intermediate density and short fibers are present in regio inferior, whereas the density of puncta and the number of fibers are higher, the latter forming a plexus, in regio superior. *Stratum radiatum* contains a few, large, stellate cell bodies in regio inferior and occasionally small, fusiform cell bodies, resembling vertical nonpyramidal cells, in regio superior. A few fibers are also present. The *layer of mossy fibers* is characterized by fibers traversing the layer. In the *pyramidal cell layer*, occasional stellate cell bodies are present in the deep part of the layer at the transition between regio inferior and regio superior and near the subiculum. A small number of fibers also traverse the layer. *Stratum oriens* is occupied by a large number of cell bodies, particularly in regio superior. The majority of these are stellate, but fusiform cell bodies, resembling horizontal nonpyramidal cells, occupy the deepest part of the layer. A few fibers are also seen. In the *alveus*, cell bodies are frequently seen displaced from stratum oriens.

In the *subiculum* (IV, Figs. 2b, 3b, 17, 18), the *plexiform layer* contains several cell bodies in the deep part of the layer near regio superior and fewer cell bodies towards the presubiculum. Puncta of high density and a plexus of fibers are present near regio superior in the superficial part of the layer, whereas the deep part is occupied by a less dense network of fibers. Towards the presubiculum, the density of puncta is smaller. The *cell layer* contains many stellate or fusiform cell bodies near regio superior and fewer, smaller cell bodies towards the presubiculum. A network of fibers is seen throughout the layer, being particularly prominent towards regio superior.

Neuropeptide Y-like immunoreactivity (NPY). The NPY staining pattern is dominated by an abundance of intensely stained fibers and fewer, occasionally weakly stained nerve cell bodies and puncta. In the *dentate area* (IV, Figs. 4b, 5b, 19), the *molecular layer* is characterized by a few, small cell bodies in the inner third of the layer, resembling molecular layer basket cells. Puncta of low density and an abundance of fibers are seen in the outer third of the layer, whereas the number of fibers is smaller in the remaining part of the layer. In the *granule cell layer*, a large number of small cell bodies is seen in the deep part of the layer, resembling pyramidal, horizontal, and fusiform basket cells. A few cell bodies are additionally seen in the superficial part of the layer, resembling inverted fusiform basket cells. Fibers are also seen traversing the layer. The *hilus* is characterized by a few stellate cell bodies located in the deep part of the outer hilar cell layer, the inner plexiform layer, and the superficial part of the inner hilar cell layer. A large number of fibers form a very dense plexus in the outer plexiform layer and outer hilar cell layer, and a less dense plexus in the inner plexiform layer and inner hilar cell layer.

In the *hippocampus proper* (IV, Figs. 4b, 5b, 24, 27), *stratum moleculare* is characterized by puncta of low density which in regio superior, particularly near the subiculum, occupy a narrow rim towards stratum radiatum. Fibers are present in small numbers in regio inferior, increasing in number towards regio superior where a dense plexus is found. This plexus furthermore increases in density towards the subiculum. *Stratum radiatum* is occupied by a few triangular or stellate cell bodies in regio inferior and a few fusiform cell bodies, resembling vertical nonpyramidal cells, in regio superior. A few fibers are also present, increasing in number towards the subiculum. The *layer of mossy fibers* is characterized by several fibers which occasionally extend into stratum radiatum and the pyramidal cell layer. In the *pyramidal cell layer*, a few triangular or stellate cell bodies are present in the deep part of the layer near regio superior. Few fibers are also present in the layer. *Stratum oriens* contains several cell bodies. Most of these are triangular or stellate, although a few fusiform cell bodies, resembling horizontal nonpyramidal cells, are present in the deep part of the layer. In the *alveus*, a few cell bodies are seen displaced from stratum oriens.

In the *subiculum* (IV, Figs. 4b, 5b, 28), the *plexiform layer* contains a few large stellate cells at the border towards the cell layer. Puncta are present in small numbers adjacent to regio superior and decreasing in density towards the presubiculum. Fibers form a very dense plexus in the superficial half of the layer, increasing in density towards the presubiculum, and a less dense plexus in the deep half of the layer. The *cell layer* contains several small cell bodies and a plexus of fibers.

Cholecystokinin-like immunoreactivity (CCK). The CCK staining pattern is characterized by numerous, usually intensely stained nerve cell bodies and fine puncta, whereas fibers are only occasionally observed. In the *dentate area* (V, Figs. 1b, 8), the *molecular layer* contains a few stellate or fusiform cell bodies. Puncta of low density occupy the inner third of the layer and single, thick fibers are occasionally seen. In the *granule cell layer*, several cell bodies are present in the deep part of the layer, resembling pyramidal, horizontal, and fusiform basket cells. In addition, a few cell bodies are seen in the superficial part of the layer, resembling inverted fusiform basket cells. Puncta of low density are also present between the granule cells in the superficial two thirds of the layer. The *hilus* is characterized by a large number of cell bodies in all parts of the hilus, resembling fusiform and stellate cells.

In the *hippocampus proper* (V, Figs. 1b, 10, 11), *stratum moleculare* contains an occasional cell body in regio inferior, whereas a few stellate cell bodies are present in regio superior, particularly at the limit towards stratum radiatum near the subiculum. Puncta are seen in low densities in regio inferior and in high densities in regio superior, particularly in the deep part of the layer. Near regio inferior, the puncta are present in a narrow rim at the limit towards stratum radiatum, increasing in width and eventually occupying the entire layer towards the subiculum. A few fibers are also present in regio inferior. *Stratum radiatum* contains several stellate or fusiform cell bodies, resembling vertical nonpyramidal cells, in the superficial half of the layer in regio inferior and a smaller number of these cell bodies in regio superior. The *layer of mossy fibers* occasionally contains a single stellate cell body. In the *pyramidal cell layer*, a few stellate cell bodies are often seen in the deep part of the layer. Puncta are present in large numbers between the pyramidal cells in regio inferior, and in smaller numbers in regio superior. *Stratum oriens* is occupied by cell bodies in small numbers in regio inferior and in higher numbers in regio superior. Some of these cell bodies are stellate, but others, particularly in the deep part of the layer, are fusiform, resembling horizontal nonpyramidal cells. Puncta are also present in small numbers in regio superior. The *alveus* contains a few cell bodies displaced from stratum oriens.

In the *subiculum* (V, Figs. 1b, 12, 13), the *plexiform layer* is characterized by several, stellate cell bodies, particularly in the deep half of the layer. Puncta are present in low densities in the superficial half of the layer, and in much higher densities in the deep half of the layer. Towards the presubiculum, the puncta gradually disappear. In the *cell layer*, several cell bodies are seen, particularly in the deep part of the layer near regio superior. Puncta are present in moderate numbers near regio superior, but gradually decrease in number towards the presubiculum, except at the limit towards the plexiform layer.

Enkephalin-like immunoreactivity (ENK). The ENK staining pattern is characterized by a very small number of faintly stained nerve cell bodies and fine fibers. Stained puncta appear very fine and distributed in a characteristic pattern. In the *dentate area* (V, Figs. 2b, 14), the *molecular layer* is characterized by an abundance of fine puncta in the inner third of the layer with the highest density in the outer part towards the unstained outer two thirds of the layer and decreasing in density towards the granule cell layer. A few fibers are also occasionally encountered. In the *granule cell layer*, a single cell body is only occasionally seen, whereas puncta are present in abundant numbers between the granule cells in the most superficial part of the layer. Fibers are encountered occasionally. The *hilus* contains a few cell bodies in the outer hilar cell layer, the inner plexiform layer, and the inner hilar cell layer, resembling fusiform or stellate cells. Puncta of moderate density surround some of the hilar neurons in the outer hilar cell layer, and a few fibers are seen in the outer plexiform layer, the outer hilar cell layer, and the inner plexiform layer.

In the *hippocampus proper* (V, Figs. 2b, 16, 17), *stratum moleculare* is characterized by a few cell bodies in regio superior. Puncta of low density form a narrow rim in the deepest part of the layer towards stratum radiatum in regio superior. Near the subiculum, this rim gradually increases in width. Many short fibers are seen in regio inferior. *Stratum radiatum* contains a few cell bodies in regio superior near the subiculum. Several, rather thick fibers are present in the deep part of the layer in the part of regio inferior near regio superior. Very long fibers are also occasionally seen in regio superior near the subiculum. In the *layer of mossy fibers*, puncta of moderate density form a demarcation of the layer against stratum radiatum near regio superior. The *pyramidal cell layer* is characterized by puncta and fibers in the deep part of the layer in the part of regio inferior near regio superior, whereas the layer appears unstained in regio superior. *Stratum oriens* contains a few cell bodies in the deep part of the layer, resembling horizontal nonpyramidal cells. Towards the subiculum, a few cell bodies, resembling deep subicular pyramidal cells, appear in the deep half of the layer. A few fibers are also seen in regio inferior, whereas stained puncta of low density are present in the deep part of the layer in regio superior, increasing in density towards the subiculum. The *alveus* contains a few cell bodies displaced from stratum oriens.

In the *subiculum* (V, Figs. 2b, 18), the *plexiform layer* contains a few stellate cell bodies in the deepest part of the layer near regio superior. Puncta of low density are present in the superficial half of the layer, whereas the number of puncta is higher in the deep half of the layer. A few fibers are also present in the superficial half of the layer. The *cell layer* is characterized by the presence of numerous pyramidal cell bodies in the deep third of the layer near regio superior. These cells display a characteristic staining which extends into the apical dendrites for some distance and the cells probably represent subicular pyramidal cells. Other cell bodies without staining of dendrites are present in the remaining part of the layer. Puncta of medium density are seen in the deep part of the layer.

Substance P-like immunoreactivity (SP). The SP staining pattern is dominated by a characteristic distribution of stained puncta, whereas stained nerve cell bodies and fibers are few in number and faintly stained. In the *dentate area* (V, Figs. 3b, 19), the *molecular layer* is occupied by puncta of low density and a few fibers in the inner third of the layer, and the *granule cell layer* is occasionally traversed by single fibers. In the *hilus*, a few cell bodies are present in the outer hilar cell layer, the inner plexiform layer, and the inner hilar cell layer, resembling fusiform and stellate cells. Puncta are present in very large numbers, particularly in the outer hilar cell layer where they form large elements of fused puncta surrounding the large hilar neurons, hence resembling axosomatic terminals. Only few puncta are seen in the outer plexiform layer and inner plexiform layer, whereas the inner hilar cell layer contains many puncta distributed in a reticular pattern between the hilar cells and converging towards the hippocampal layer of mossy fibers, resembling mossy fiber terminals. A small number of fibers are also seen throughout the hilus.

In the *hippocampus proper* (V, 3b, 21, 22), *stratum moleculare* appears unstained in regio inferior, whereas puncta of low density and a few fibers are present in regio superior. Near the subiculum, the density of puncta increases, forming a narrow rim towards stratum radiatum, and the number of fibers increases, too. *Stratum radiatum* contains a few cell bodies. Puncta and fibers are present in small numbers in regio inferior, increasing in number in regio superior. The *layer of mossy fibers* is characterized by a very large number of large elements of fused puncta, resembling mossy fiber giant boutons. The elements are slightly more numerous near regio superior. In the *pyramidal cell layer*, single cell bodies are occasionally seen in the deep part of the layer. Fibers are also seen traversing the layer, particularly in regio superior. *Stratum oriens* contains only few cell bodies in regio inferior, but a large number of cell bodies in regio superior, resembling horizontal nonpyramidal cells. Puncta of low density are also seen, whereas fibers appear in particularly high numbers in the deep half of the layer in regio superior. The *alveus* occasionally contains cell bodies displaced from stratum oriens.

In the *subiculum* (V, Figs. 3b, 23), the *plexiform layer* is characterized by puncta of very low density in the superficial half of the layer, and a much larger number of puncta in the deep half of the layer together with many fibers. The *cell layer* contains several stellate cell bodies in the deep half of the layer near regio superior, and a large number of puncta and fibers. The number of puncta and fibers decreases towards the presubiculum.

The distribution of the neuropeptides examined in the present studies has been reported in a large variety of mammals, including rats, mice, voles, hamsters, guinea pigs, hedgehogs, rabbits, squirrels, sheep, cats, tree shrews, monkeys, and humans (see references in IV and V). Comparison of the distribution of neuropeptides in these species has shown pronounced similarities in both the SS and NPY systems in the hippocampal region, suggesting a high degree of conservation of these systems throughout phylogeny, whereas each of the CCK, ENK, and SP systems shows considerable interspecies variation in the hippocampal region (*Gall* 1990). The results of the present studies in the pig hippocampus confirm this general view.

The distribution of SS and NPY nerve cell bodies and terminals in the pig hippocampus shows a high degree of resemblance to that of other mammals. However, more detailed analysis reveals more subtle species specific differences in the distribution of stained fibers, particularly in the dentate area and the layer of mossy fibers. In the dentate area of the pig, SS and NPY fibers are present in large numbers, forming fiber plexuses in the outer third of the dentate molecular layer as well as in the outer plexiform layer and outer hilar cell layer of the dentate hilus. A comparison of SS in the dentate area of rats, monkeys (*Macaca fascicularis*), and humans (*Amaral et al.* 1988) showed a greater density of fiber and terminal labelling in the dentate molecular layer of monkeys and humans than of rats, and a substantially higher number of labelled fibers in the inner third of the human molecular layer than seen in the monkey. In addition, the dentate hilus of the monkey (*Macaca fascicularis*) contains many SS fibers which are most dense in the "pauci-cellular zone" adjacent to the granule cell layer (*Bakst et al.* 1985), whereas the human dentate hilus contains a heterogeneous meshwork of SS fibers (*Chan-Palay* 1987; *Amaral et al.* 1988). SS fibers are not described in the dentate hilus of other species. NPY fibers, on the other hand, are present in the outer part of the dentate molecular layer of rats and monkeys (*Cynomolgus*) (*Köhler et al.* 1986) and humans (*Chan-Palay et al.* 1986a; *Lotstra et al.* 1989), as well as in the human dentate hilus, there forming a meshwork of scattered fibers (*Chan-Palay et al.* 1986a; *Lotstra et al.* 1989). Taken together, the distribution of SS fibers in the dentate hilus of the pig resembles that of the monkey (*Macaca fascicularis*) the most, whereas the distribution of NPY fibers in the pig dentate hilus indicates that the pig possesses a much more elaborate system of NPY fibers in the hilus than other species. The identical localization of SS and NPY fiber plexuses in the outer plexiform layer and outer hilar cell layer of the pig dentate hilus coincides with the previously mentioned presence of very high intensity of Timm staining observed in the outer hilar cell layer. A similar correspondence is seen between the Timm staining pattern and the localization of SS fibers in the monkey dentate hilus, in that the highest intensity of Timm staining in the dentate hilus of the monkey (*Macaca mulatta*) is present in the polymorphic zone (*Rosene and van Hoesen* 1987) corresponding to the above mentioned localization of the high density of SS fibers in a closely related monkey (*Macaca fascicularis*) (*Bakst et al.* 1985). The layer of mossy fibers of the pig contains both SS and NPY fibers. SS fibers are likewise present in small numbers in the layer of mossy fibers in the monkey (*Macaca fascicularis*) (*Bakst et al.* 1985), but not in other species, whereas NPY fibers are not previously described in the layer of mossy fibers in any of the other species studied so far.

The distribution of CCK, ENK and SP nerve cell bodies in the pig hippocampus largely corresponds with observations in other mammals. Whereas the distribution of CCK terminals in the pig hippocampus in many ways resembles that of other mammals, the distribution of both ENK and SP terminals in the pig hippocampus differs markedly from that observed in other mammals. Interspecies variability in the distribution of CCK, ENK, and SP terminals is best illustrated in relation to the termination of afferent projections, which is particularly well known in the rodent hippocampus (Fig. 1), but not yet described in pigs. CCK puncta in the pig hippocampus are found in the inner third of the dentate molecular layer, corresponding to the termination of the commissural-associational system (CA) of the rat hippocampus (*Zimmer* 1971; *Laurberg and Sørensen* 1981), and in the middle third of the dentate molecular layer and the deep part of stratum moleculare of the hippocampal regio inferior and regio superior, corresponding to the termination of the medial perforant path (MPP) and medial temporoammonic tract (MTA) of the rat hippocampus (*Hjorth-Simonsen and Jeune* 1972; *Steward*

1976), whereas the dentate hilus and the layer of mossy fibers in the hippocampal regio inferior, forming the mossy fiber system (MF) of the rat hippocampus, appear unstained. For comparison, the CA system likewise appears stained in the mouse (*Gall et al.* 1986; *Fredens et al.* 1987), rat (*Stengaard-Pedersen et al.* 1983; *Fredens et al.* 1987), gerbil, cat, monkey (*Gall* 1990), and humans (*Lotstra and Vanderhaeghen* 1987), but is unstained in the hedgehog (*Stengaard-Pedersen et al.* 1983), guinea pig (*Stengaard-Pedersen et al.* 1983; *Gall* 1984), and rabbit (*Gall* 1990). The MPP-MTA system is also stained in the mouse (*Gall et al.* 1986), rat (*Stengaard-Pedersen et al.* 1983; *Fredens et al.* 1984), guinea pig (*Gall* 1984), gerbil, rabbit, cat, monkey (*Gall* 1990), and humans (*Lotstra and Vanderhaeghen* 1987), but not in the hedgehog (*Stengaard-Pedersen et al.* 1983). The MF system is likewise unstained in the rat (*Stengaard-Pedersen et al.* 1983), rabbit, cat, (*Gall* 1990), and humans (*Lotstra and Vanderhaeghen* 1987), but appears stained in the mouse (*Gall et al.* 1986), guinea pig (*Stengaard-Pedersen et al.* 1983; *Gall* 1984), hedgehog (*Stengaard-Pedersen et al.* 1983), gerbil, and monkey (*Gall* 1990). The most notable features of the distribution of ENK puncta in the pig hippocampus in relation to other species are the presence of puncta in the inner third of the dentate molecular layer, corresponding to the CA system, and the absence of puncta in the dentate hilus and the layer of mossy fibers, corresponding to the MF system. In other species examined, staining of the CA system is not reported, whereas staining of the MF system is found in all other species except humans. Furthermore, staining of the outer third of the dentate molecular layer, the superficial part of stratum moleculare of the hippocampal regio inferior, and stratum moleculare of the hippocampal regio superior, corresponding to the termination of the lateral perforant path (LPP) and lateral temporoammonic tract (LTA) of the rat hippocampus (*Hjorth-Simonsen* 1972; *Hjorth-Simonsen and Jeune* 1972; *Steward* 1976), is absent in the pig as well as in the hedgehog (*Stengaard-Pedersen et al.* 1983) and tree shrew (*Fitzpatrick and Johnson* 1981), but appears stained in the rat (*Gall et al.* 1981; *Stengaard-Pedersen et al.* 1983; *Fredens et al.* 1984; *McLean et al.* 1987), hamster (*McLean et al.* 1987), and monkey (*Macaca fascicularis*) (*Gall* 1990). In the mouse (*Gall* 1988; *van Daal et al.* 1989), guinea pig (*Tielen et al.* 1982), and cat (*Gall* 1990), puncta are seen in both the outer and middle thirds of the dentate molecular layer. Finally, the dentate molecular layer of the squirrel is characterized by a thin layer of stained puncta between the granule cell layer and the inner third of the molecular layer (*McLean et al.* 1987), corresponding to the termination of afferents from the supramammillary hypothalamic nucleus (SH system) in rats and guinea pigs (*Haglund et al.* 1984; *Gall and Selawski* 1984). The distribution of SP puncta in the pig hippocampus differs markedly from other species, the most conspicuous difference being the staining of the dentate hilus and the layer of mossy fibers, corresponding to the MF system, in the pig. In humans, a similar type of staining is present in the dentate hilus (*Sakamoto et al.* 1987), whereas staining of the MF system is absent from all other species studied. Unlike the pig, stained fibers are present in the inner third of the dentate molecular layer and the superficial part of the granule cell layer, possibly corrresponding to the SH system, in the guinea pig (*Gall and Selawski* 1984), squirrel (*Gall* 1990), cat (*Vincent et al.* 1981; *Ino et al.* 1988; *Yanagihara and Niimi* 1989), monkey [*Macaca fuscata fuscata* (*Iritani et al.* 1989), *Macaca fascicularis* and *Saimiri sciureus* (*Gall* 1990)], and humans (*Del Fiacco et al.* 1987; *Sakamoto et al.* 1987; *Lotstra et al.* 1988; *Quigley and Kowall* 1991).

The distribution of each of the neuropeptides in the pig hippocampus displays significant septotemporal variation. A similar variation is seen in the hippocampus of other mammals, the temporal part of the hippocampus being generally more "peptide-rich" than the more septal part (*Gall* 1990). This variation probably reflects septotemporal differences in the organization of intrinsic and extrinsic connections of the hippocampus as described in detail by *Witter* (1986), and should be taken into account when evaluating data in future experimental studies.

Several of the neuropeptides are known to be co-localized with GABA or GAD in distinct subpopulations of hippocampal nongranule and nonpyramidal cells. The majority (91%) of SS nerve cell bodies in the rat hippocampus are GABAergic (*Schmechel et al.* 1984; *Somogyi et al.* 1984; *Kosaka et al.* 1988), and almost all CCK nerve cell bodies are estimated to be GABAergic, while only about 10% of the GABAergic nerve cell bodies contain CCK, depending on the localization (*Kosaka et al.* 1985). Vasoactive intestinal polypeptide (VIP) likewise is co-localized with GAD (*Kosaka et al.* 1985). SS and NPY furthermore show a variable degree of co-localization in the different hippocampal subfields (*Köhler et al.* 1987; *Chan-Palay* 1987).

The functional significance of neuropeptides in hippocampal physiology is not fully understood. Neuropeptides differ from the classical neurotransmitters in that they are active in extremely low concentrations and with extremely high potency, display low-affinity binding to receptors and a low rate of synthesis, and have long-term effects (*Shepherd* 1988). Neuropeptides are believed to play a neuromodulatory role in that they modify the known actions of classical neurotransmitters, act to block the release of a given neurotransmitter via their release at presynaptic endings on the terminals releasing that transmitter, or alter the turnover of other neurotransmitters (*Krieger* 1983).

3.4 Calcium-Binding Proteins (VI)

Like the neuropeptides, the calcium-binding proteins calbindin-D 28k (CaBP) and parvalbumin (PV) were visualized using immunocytochemistry, and the resulting staining likewise includes immunoreactive nerve cell bodies, puncta, and fibers. The following summary follows the strategy used for the neuropeptides.

Calbindin-D 28k (CaBP). In the *dentate area* (VI, Figs. 4b, 11, 12), the *molecular layer* is characterized by many small cell bodies in the outer third of the layer and a few stellate cell bodies in the intermediate third of the layer. Puncta of moderate density are present in the inner third of the layer, whereas fibers are seen in large numbers in the outer third of the layer and in small numbers in the inner third of the layer. In the *granule cell layer*, a very large number of puncta are present between the granule cells in the most superficial part of the layer. The *hilus* contains a few stellate cell bodies in the outer plexiform layer, the outer hilar cell layer, and the inner hilar cell layer, whereas fibers are present in moderate numbers in the outer plexiform layer and outer hilar cell layer.

In the *hippocampus proper* (VI, Figs. 4b, 6, 7, 8), *stratum moleculare* contains many small cell bodies. Puncta of high density are present throughout the layer, increasing in density towards the subiculum. A large number of fibers are additionally seen. *Stratum radiatum* is characterized by a few stellate and fusiform cell bodies, resembling vertical nonpyramidal cells, and moderate numbers of long fibers. In the *layer of mossy fibers*, stellate cell bodies are occasionally seen. A narrow rim of puncta is present at the limit towards stratum radiatum and the layer is often traversed by fibers. The *pyramidal cell layer* occasionally contains small cell bodies in the deep part of the layer. Puncta are also seen between the pyramidal cells, showing particularly high density in the deep part of the layer in regio inferior. In *stratum oriens*, several large stellate cell bodies, resembling horizontal nonpyramidal cells, are present, as well as moderate numbers of fibers. The *alveus* contains a small number of fibers.

In the *subiculum* (VI, Figs. 4b, 5), the *plexiform layer* is characterized by stellate cell bodies and a very high number of fibers, particularly in the superficial half of the layer. The *cell layer* contains a large number of intensely stained subicular pyramidal cells whose apical dendrites extend into the plexiform layer. A very high density of puncta is also seen in the layer.

Parvalbumin (PV). In the *dentate area* (VI, Figs. 4c, 17, 18), the *molecular layer* contains puncta of low density in the inner third of the layer as well as a small number of fibers. The *granule cell layer* is characterized by cell bodies located in the deep part of the layer, resembling horizontal, pyramidal, and fusiform basket cells, as well as a large number of puncta between the granule cells. In the *hilus*, many stellate cell bodies are seen in the outer plexiform layer and the outer hilar cell layer, whereas the inner hilar cell layer only contains a few cell bodies. A small number of fibers are additionally seen in the outer plexiform layer and outer hilar cell layer.

In the *hippocampus proper* (VI, Figs. 4c, 13, 14), *stratum moleculare* is devoid of immunoreactivity. *Stratum radiatum* occasionally contains cell bodies, resembling vertical nonpyramidal cells. In the *layer of mossy fibers*, single cell bodies are occasionally seen. The *pyramidal cell layer* is characterized by a few cell bodies in the deep part of the layer and puncta between the pyramidal cells showing higher dentity in regio inferior than in regio superior. *Stratum oriens* contains several stellate cell bodies, resembling horizontal nonpyramidal cells, and a few fibers. In the *alveus*, a few fibers are present.

In the *subiculum* (VI, Fig. 4c), a few cell bodies are seen in the deep part of the *cell layer*. The remaining part of the subiculum appears unstained.

The distribution of CaBP and PV has been described in the hippocampal region of rats (*Jande et al.* 1981; *Baimbridge and Miller* 1982; *Miller and Baimbridge* 1983; *Rami et al.* 1987; *Heizmann and Celio* 1987; *Kosaka et al.* 1987; *Katsumaru et al.* 1988; *Sloviter* 1989b; *Kamphuis et al.* 1989; *Nitsch et al.* 1990; *Ribak et al.* 1990; *Gulyás et al.* 1991), guinea pigs (*Rami et al.* 1987), European hedgehogs (*Rami et al.* 1987; *Ferrer et al.* 1992), monkeys [*Macaca mulatta* (*Seress et al.* 1991), *Cercopithecus aethiops* (*Leranth and Ribak* 1991; *Ribak et al.* 1993), *Papio papio* (*Sloviter et al.* 1991), *Macaca fascicularis* (*Pitkänen and Amaral* 1993)], and humans (*Berchtold et al.* 1985; *Sloviter et al.* 1991; *Braak et al.* 1991; *Seress et al.* 1992). The distribution of PV nerve cell bodies and terminals in the pig hippocampus appears identical to that described in all other mammals so far studied. In contrast, the distribution of CaBP nerve cell bodies and terminals in the pig hippocampus differs fundamentally from other mammals. In rats, guinea pigs, hedgehogs, monkeys, and humans, CaBP is present in the dentate granule cells and the mossy fiber system, as well as in a subpopulation of nongranule and nonpyramidal cells. With the exception of the guinea pig, the pyramidal cells of regio superior also contain CaBP in these species. In the pig hippocampus, CaBP is absent from the dentate granule cells, the mossy fiber system, and the pyramidal cells of regio superior, whereas a subpopulation of nongranule and nonpyramidal cells contains CaBP.

Co-localization studies in rats have shown that both CaBP and PV are present in GABAergic nongranule and nonpyramidal cells. Almost all (97%) PV neurons also contain GAD, whereas only 22.4% of the GAD neurons contain PV, the latter depending on the localization (*Kosaka et al.* 1987). However, using antiserum against GABA, *Kamphuis et al.* (1989) found a much lower percentage (25%) of GABA containing PV cells in regio superior. On the other hand, the majority (81%) of CaBP nonpyramidal cells are GABAergic (*Tóth and Freund* 1992). Coexistence of CaBP and PV has been reported in stratum oriens of regio superior (9.6% of PV cells contain CaBP), but only rarely in other parts of the hippocamus (*Gulyás et al.* 1991). Coexistence of CaBP and CCK was also seen in stratum radiatum of regio inferior, where 12.5% of CaBP cells contain CCK whereas 21.2% of CCK cells contain CaBP (*Gulyás et al.* 1991).

The functional significance of calcium-binding proteins is related to their supposed role as calcium ion buffers (*Baimbridge and Miller* 1982; *Heizmann* 1984). The role of calcium ions in the control of neurotransmitter release, neuronal excitability and neuronal plasticity makes the distribution of calcium-binding proteins of general interest in neurobiology. However, the involvement of calcium ions in cell death adds to the importance of calcium-binding proteins in clinical conditions involving neuronal death. According to the calcium overload hypothesis, cell death is preceded by pathological accumulation of intracellular calcium which activates biochemical processes leading to enzymatic breakdown of proteins and lipids, malfunctioning mitochondria and energy failure (*Siesjö and Bengtsson* 1989). It has therefore been assumed that neurons containing calcium-binding proteins, and thereby having a greater capacity to buffer intracellular calcium, are more resistant to degeneration. This was supported by experimental evidence of decreased vulnerability of hippocampal neurons (mossy cells of the dentate hilus) to damage resulting from electrical stimulation following intracellular chelation of calcium (*Scharfman and Schwartzkroin* 1989). Furthermore, a positive correlation was described between the presence of at least one of the calcium-binding proteins in hippocampal neurons and their relative resistance to seizure-induced neuronal damage (*Sloviter* 1989b). Several experimental studies have been performed to elucidate the possible resistance of CaBP and PV neurons in pathological conditions (see Clinical Perspectives), and these studies have failed to show an unequivocal protective role of calcium-binding proteins. Indeed, there seems to be no consistent and systematic relationship between neuronal CaBP or PV content and ischaemic vulnerability (*Freund et al.* 1990). Rather, it can be speculated that neurons containing CaBP and PV normally require these proteins for the regulation of intracellular calcium levels in connection with neurotransmission or neuronal plasticity which employ calcium in their normal operations (*Freund et al.* 1990). For review, see *Heizmann and Braun* 1992).

3.5 Volumes of Hippocampal Subdivisions and Number of Neurons (VII)

The morphometrical analysis included estimation of the volumes of the telencephalon, fascia dentata, hilus fasciae dentatae, regio inferior, regio superior, and the subiculum and estimation of the number of neurons in the granule cell layer, hilus fasciae dentatae, the pyramidal cell layer of regio inferior and regio superior, and the cell layer of the subiculum. The mean values of the estimates of the volumes are given in VII, Table I together with the means of the coefficients of error, $\overline{CE}$, and the observed relative variation among animals, CV. In VII, Table II, the mean values of the estimates of the number of neurons are shown, as well as the means of the coefficients of error, $\overline{CE}$, and the observed relative variation among animals, CV.

In order to evaluate the quantitative descriptions with respect to their potential use in experimental studies, the implications of the variances of the individual and group estimates will be discussed. The observed relative variance of the group, CV^2 (CV = SD/mean, for the estimates in five pigs), is the sum of the inherent, or real, variance, ICV^2 (related to the fact that pigs are different), and the observed relative variance of the estimate made in individuals, $\overline{CE}^2$ (CE = SEM/mean), i.e.

$$CV^2 = ICV^2 + \overline{CE}^2$$

The mean CEs ($\overline{CE}$) for both volume and number estimates are less than 0.10 for all subdivisions (VII, Tables I and II) indicating that the described sampling schemes provide a precision of the individual estimates that is more than sufficient for studies in which the inherent biological variance is 10% of the mean of the group. With the exception of regio inferior, the $\overline{CE}^2$s for both the volume and number estimates are less than half of the CV^2s (see VII, Tables I and II for $\overline{CE}$ and CV values), indicating that in these cases most of the observed relative variance for the group, CV^2, is contributed by the inherent variance, ICV^2 (biological variation between the pigs), and not by the observed relative variance of the estimate made in individuals, $\overline{CE}^2$ (the precision of the stereological estimates). In these cases, the CV^2 is best reduced by the addition of more pigs to the group. This is not the case for the volume and number estimates made in regio inferior, where it would be more efficient to first increase the amount of sampling in each individual.

Another way to think about the precision of the methodology described here is in terms of an investigator's ability to resolve differences between group means. Under the assumption that the variances of the estimates are similar in two groups to be compared, and each group is composed of five pigs similar to those used in this study, the means of the group estimates of volume would have to differ by 10% to 22% and the estimates of neuron number would have to differ by 17% to 22% in order for the respective estimates to be considered significantly different in the statistical sense. With the exception of the limited improvements in the precision of the estimates of number and volume in regio inferior that could be achieved through more sampling in the five individuals already in the group, the most efficient way to improve the sensitivity of the stereological methodology, with regard to the comparison of group means, would be to add individuals to the groups.

It is possible, however, to further reduce the observed group variance of estimates made in this study by nonstereological means. From studies of inbred laboratory rats from the same litter and of the same age, it has been shown that the inherent biological variance is significantly less than that seen in the pigs used in this study (*West et al.* 1991). Many strains of domestic pigs are as highly inbred as laboratory rats and can be obtained from standardized environments comparable to those in which laboratory animals are raised. Through a more rigorous selection of pigs, with regard to age and environment, it should be possible to reduce inter-individual variability further and produce a higher degree of precision in the group estimates using the same number of animals and the sampling schemes used in this study.

In order to compare the volumetric data from the pig hippocampus with similar data from other species, the percentage of the telencephalic volume occupied by the hippocampus as well as the relative proportions of the hippocampal subdivisions in percentage of the total hippocampal volume are shown in VII, Figs. 7 and 8 for the pig and other species. The other species included European hedgehog (*Erinaceus europaeus*), harvest mouse (*Micromys minutus*), DBA/2J laboratory mouse (*Mus musculus*), Wistar strain albino laboratory rat (*Mus norvegicus albinus*), tree shrew (*Tupaia glis*), marmoset monkey (*Callithrix jacchus*), and humans (Homo sapiens) (*West* 1990). During mammalian evolution, most of the increase in relative brain size can be attributed to the neocortex. Although the hippocampus also increases in size, relative to body weight, during mammalian evolution (*Stephan* 1983), the increase in the size of the neocortex exceeds that of the hippocampus and the hippocampus occupies a decreasing proportion of the telencephalon. It is therefore interesting to see that the percentage of the telencephalon occupied by the hippocampus in the pig (2.56%) lies between the values obtained in humans (0.7%) and in other primates, such as tree shrew (8.5%) and marmoset (3.7%) (VII, Fig. 7). It should be noted that while our data from the pig are based on prepubertal animals (14 weeks old), the data from all other species were obtained from adult animals. At 14 weeks of age, the pig brain has reached 90% of its adult size (*van Eerdenburg et al.* 1990) and we believe that the relationship between the volumes of the hippocampus and the telencephalon does not change significantly during puberty. In Fig. 8, the relative proportions of the subdivisions of the hippocampus are shown as a percentage of the total volume of the hippocampus for the pig, as well as for the species mentioned above (*West* 1990). In the pig, the percentages of the subdivisions are: fascia dentata (16%), hilus fasciae dentatae (12%), regio inferior (23%), regio superior (33%), and subiculum (16%). The most notable feature of the pig hippocampus is the relatively large hilus which occupies a larger percentage of the total volume of the hippocampus (12%) than it does in humans (9%). As mentioned previously, the hilus of the pig is highly laminar, resembling that of primates, and it can be argued that only the outer hilar cells belong to the hilus, while the inner hilar cell layer should be regarded as modified pyramidal cells of the hippocampal regio inferior. In the present quantitative study, the inner hilar cell layer is included in the hilus, following the strategy of the descriptive studies and allowing comparisons with the previous data from other species. Comparison of the number of neurons in the hippocampal subdivisions of the pig with similar data from other species is more limited, because similar data so far only exist for rats (*West et al.* 1991) and humans (*West and Gundersen* 1990). The intraspecies relationship between the volume and the number of neurons in homologous hippocampal subdivisions is shown in VII, Fig. 9, in which the log of the mean number of neurons is plotted as a function of the log of the mean volume of the specific subdivisions in domestic pigs, rats, and humans. For all subdivisions, there is a significant positive nonlinear correlation between the number of neurons and the volume of the subdivision. The regression coefficients for this relationship in the different subdivisions are: fascia dentata, 0.70; hilus fasciae dentatae, 0.74; regio inferior, 0.64; regio superior, 0.74; subiculum, 0.60; combined hilus and regio inferior, 0.69. On the average, the difference in the number of neurons in homologous subdivisions is proportional to the 0.68 power of the difference in volume.

$$N \sim V^{0.68}$$

That is, for every three fold increase in volume there is roughly a two fold increase in the number of neurons. This suggests an isomorphic transformation of hippocampal homologues during speciation with the implication that the number of neurons per radial unit is maintained and that the total number of neurons is augmented during speciation by the addition of radial units that contain a constant number of neurons. This in turn implies that the output of a specific region, i.e. the number of discrete channels, scales essentially like a surface of an object that changes in size but not shape, and that the input, i.e. the number of synapses, scales as a function of the volume in that their number per unit volume remains relatively constant across species lines (see *West* 1990). An isomorphic transformation has the additional consequence that the number of synapses per neuron scales in proportion to the height of the radial unit or cortical thickness, that is, it scales roughly in proportion to the 1/3 power of the volume.

4. CLINICAL PERSPECTIVES

In the following, some of the pathological findings in the hippocampus associated with temporal lobe epilepsy, hypoxic-ischaemic damage, and Alzheimer's disease will be mentioned briefly with special reference to neuropeptides and calcium-binding proteins.

Among the pathological findings observed in hippocampi from patients suffering from temporal lobe epilepsy as well as in experimental epilepsy models are synaptic rearrangements in the dentate gyrus and a selective loss of neuropeptide-containing nerve cell bodies. The synaptic rearrangements include sprouting of mossy fibers into the granule cell layer and inner third of the molecular layer in epileptic patients (*Sutula et al.* 1989; *Houser et al.* 1990), electrically kindled rats (*Sutula et al.* 1988; *Cavazos et al.* 1991), and rats treated with kainic acid (*Tauck and Nadler* 1985) and pentylenetetrazol (*Golarai et al.* 1992). In normal rats, recurrent mossy fibers form synapses with nongranule cells (basket cells) (*Ribak and Peterson* 1991). These basket cells are GABAergic inhibitory neurons responsible for feedback and feedforward inhibition of granule cells. However, sprouted mossy fibers form synapses with granule cells following lesions (*Frotscher and Zimmer* 1983), and it has therefore been hypothesized that in case of severe seizures associated with cell loss and sprouting of mossy fibers, the sprouted fibers form synapses with granule cells (*Ribak and Peterson* 1991). This would increase recurrent excitation of the granule cells and may thus contribute to the development of abnormal excitability in epileptic hippocampi. Other findings in patients with temporal lobe epilepsy include a selective loss of SS and NPY hilar neurons and axonal sprouting from other hilar NPY neurons into the dentate molecular layer (*de Lanerolle et al.* 1989; *Robbins et al.* 1991), while GABAergic neurons (*Babb et al.* 1989) and CaBP and PV neurons (*Sloviter et al.* 1991) seem to survive. Experimental studies of the pathophysiological changes in the hippocampus have shown similar results, i.e. a selective loss of SS and NPY neurons, but survival of CCK, VIP, and GABAergic neurons (*Sloviter* 1987, 1991), and it has been proposed that seizure induced loss of hilar neurons that normally excite inhibitory basket cells plays a role in the pathophysiology of temporal lobe epilepsy (*Sloviter* 1987, 1991). Others have, however, reported an increase in SS of dentate hilar cells and their projections into the molecular layer of electrically kindled rats (*Orzi et al.* 1990; *Wanscher et al.* 1990) and increased NPY in the layer of mossy fibers in rats following kainic acid induced seizures and pentylenetetrazol kindling (*Marksteiner et al.* 1990). The discrepancies between the results of the latter studies and those of *Sloviter* (1987, 1991) might be explained by differences in the amount of stimulation used to elicit the seizures. In other studies, a consistent increase in ENK in the mossy fiber system and the entorhinal temporoammonic and perforant path projections was observed following either intracerebral injection of kainic acid (*McGinty et al.* 1983; *Kanamatsu et al.* 1986b), electrical stimulation (*Kanamatsu et al.* 1986a; *Hong et al.* 1985; *Wanscher et al.* 1990), or electrolytic lesions in the dentate hilus (*White et al.* 1987; *Gall* 1988) to induce hippocampal seizures or kindling. In addition, a decrease in CCK was observed in the mossy fiber system (*Gall* 1988). Electrical stimulation and kindling of rats result in a variety of changes in the number of CaBP and PV cells in the hippocampus, depending on which stimulation paradigm is used. Stimulation of the perforant path causes a reduction in a subpopulation of GABAergic nongranule cells in the dentate area (basket cells) which are immunoreactive to PV, whereas CaBP in granule cells is unchanged (*Sloviter* 1991). However, electrical kindling of the perforant path or the commissural fibers results in decreased CaBP levels in granule cells and mossy fibers (*Miller and Baimbridge* 1983; *Baimbridge et al.* 1985), whereas electrical kindling of the commissural fibers results in an increased number of PV neurons (*Kamphuis et al.* 1989).

The pathological changes in the hippocampus of experimental animals following central ischaemia include, among others, a loss of pyramidal cells in regio superior, preceded by a loss of SS hilar neurons (*Johansen et al.* 1987), and a loss of NPY neurons in the dentate hilus as well as in the hippocampal regio superior and regio inferior (*Johansen and O'Hare* 1989). In relation to this it was hypothesized that the ischaemia induced loss of hilar SS neurons that innervate inhibitory GABAergic neurons in the dentate area may induce hyperactivity in the hippocampus, eventually damaging the pyramidal cells in regio superior (*Johansen et al.* 1987). More recent studies, however, do suggest that this hypothesis is far too simplified, in that no hyperactivity could be demonstrated in postischaemic hippocampi (*Johansen et al.* 1991), whereas inhibition of normal hippocampal activity offered some protection against ischaemic damage (*Johansen and Diemer* 1991). After transient ischaemia (*Johansen et al.* 1990), the number and staining intensity of PV cells and fibers in the hippocampal regio superior and regio inferior and in the dentate hilus decrease, whereas PV in terminal fields is unchanged. However, PV later reappears, first in somata, then in fibers (*Johansen et al.* 1990). Others have reported a partial loss of PV nonpyramidal cells in regio superior accompanying a complete loss of pyramidal cells in regio superior, but unchanged PV cells, fibers, and terminal fields in regio inferior and the dentate area (*Freund et al.* 1990). CaBP, on the other hand, is permanently lost from pyramidal cells of regio superior, whereas CaBP in nongranule and nonpyramidal cells and in the dentate granule cells and mossy fibers is unchanged (*Freund et al.* 1990; *Johansen et al.* 1990).

Alzheimer's disease is characterized by histopathological changes involving SS, NPY, and SP neurons in the hippocampus and neocortex. Hippocampal SS neurons and axons are reduced in numbers, particularly in the dentate hilus, regio superior, and entorhinal and perirhinal cortices (*Chan-Palay* 1987), whereas NPY neurons and axons are most severely affected in the dentate hilus, regio superior, parasubiculum, and entorhinal cortex (*Chan-Palay et al.* 1986b). Furthermore, SS and NPY neurons are equally severely affected in the dentate area and regio superior, whereas a numerically higher survival is seen of NPY than SS neurons in the cortical areas. Neurons with coexistence of SS and NPY appear not to be better protected against pathological changes than neurons containing only SS (*Chan-Palay* 1987). In addition, SP appear to be colocalized with SS in plaques in the hippocampus and amygdala, but not in the remaining part of the neocortex (*Armstrong et al.* 1989). Furthermore, SP is generally reduced in both the hippocampus and neocortex in patients suffering from either senile dementia or Alzheimer's disease as compared to controls (*Bouras et al.* 1990), and a significant loss of staining intensity of both SP perikarya, terminals, and fibers is seen in the dentate gyrus, whereas dystrophic SP neurons are present in the hippocampus proper (*Quigley and Kowall* 1991). Finally, a significant loss of PV neurons is seen in the frontal and temporal cortices as well as a reduction in the size of PV neurons in the temporal cortex of Alzheimer's disease patients (*Arai et al.* 1987). CaBP neurons in frontal, temporal and parietal cortices are likewise reduced in number and size in Alzheimer's disease patients (*Ichimiya et al.* 1988).

The findings of this study of the hippocampal region of the domestic pig indicate that the pig possesses a fairly large dentate area with clear resemblance to that of primates. In view of the central role of the dentate area in the pathogenesis of temporal lobe epilepsy and hypoxic-ischaemic damage, it is tempting to assume that the domestic pig may prove valuable as an alternative experimental model for these clinical conditions affecting the hippocampus. Recently, the pig has proven useful as experimental model for Parkinson's disease. Preliminary results have shown altered behaviour (hypokinesia and rigidity) (*Møller et al.* in preparation) and a loss of dopaminergic neurons in the substantia nigra in minipigs exposed to MPTP (*Møller and Østergaard*, personal communication). Future experimental studies in pigs will prove whether this animal can be used as experimental model for clinical conditions affecting the hippocampus.

5. CONCLUSIONS

The present study was undertaken with the purpose of providing a) a comparative description of the hippocampal region of the domestic pig (*Sus scrofa domesticus*) with reference to other mammalian species previously studied, and b) baseline observations for comparison with future experimental pathophysiological studies using the domestic pig as experimental model for hippocampus related clinical conditions such as temporal lobe epilepsy, hypoxic-ischaemic neuronal damage, and Alzheimer's disease. The study includes a description of the hippocampal subdivisions as defined by the Timm staining pattern, visualizing zinc in synaptic vesicles. Furthermore, the distribution of the neuropeptides somatostatin, neuropeptide Y, cholecystokinin, enkephalin, and substance P and the calcium-binding proteins calbindin-D 28k and parvalbumin, all known to be involved in hippocampal pathology, is described. Finally, an estimation of the size of the hippocampal subdivisions and the number of neurons in these is obtained using stereological techniques.

The results indicate that the overall organization of the pig hippocampus, as displayed by the general cytoarchitecture and the Timm staining pattern, is fundamentally similar to that of other mammals. Of particular interest is the highly laminated dentate hilus which shows a clear resemblance to that of primates and occupy a larger percentage of the total volume of the hippocampus than it does in other species. The distribution of somatostatin, neuropeptide Y, and cholecystokinin in the pig hippocampus in general resembles that of previously described mammals, whereas the distribution of enkephalin and substance P differs markedly from other species, in that, unlike all other species so far studied, enkephalin is absent from the mossy fiber system of the pig hippocampus while substance P is present in the mossy fiber system of the pig hippocampus. Finally, the distribution of parvalbumin in the pig hippocampus generally resembles that of previously studied mammals, whereas calbindin-D 28k, unlike other mammals, is absent from the dentate granule cells and the mossy fiber system as well as the pyramidal cells of the pig hippocampus.

In view of the central role of the dentate area in the pathogenesis of temporal lobe epilepsy and hypoxic-ischaemic neuronal damage, it is tempting to assume that the pig with its fairly large dentate area with clear resemblance to that of primates may prove valuable as an alternative experimental model for these clinical conditions affecting the hippocampus.

6. DANISH SUMMARY

Formålet med nærværende undersøgelse har været at foretage en beskrivelse af hippocampusregionen hos tamsvin (*Sus scrofa domesticus*) med henblik på dels at sammenligne denne fylogenetisk set gamle del af hjernen hos svin med andre pattedyr, dels at danne basis for fremtidig etablering af dyreforsøgsmodeller på svin for temporallaps epilepsi, hypoxisk-iskæmisk neurondød og Alzheimers sygdom, som alle involverer hippocampusregionen. Undersøgelsen omfatter en beskrivelse af de forskellige områder af hippocampusregionen, som de fremtræder med Timms farvemetode. Desuden er fordelingen af neuropeptiderne somatostatin, neuropeptid Y, cholecystokinin, enkephalin og substans P og af de calciumbindende proteiner calbindin-D 28k og parvalbumin, der alle er involveret ved patologiske tilstande i hippocampusregionen, beskrevet. Endelig er der foretaget en estimering af størrelsen af de hippocampale områder og antallet af neuroner i disse.

Resultaterne viser, at den generelle opbygning (cytoarkitektur og inddeling i underområder) af hippocampusregionen hos svin er grundlæggende identisk med andre pattedyrs hippocampus. Det fremhæves især, at hilus fasciae dentatae hos svin fremtræder tydeligt lagdelt som hos primater og optager en større procentdel af det samlede volumen af hippocampus end hos andre pattedyr. Fordelingen af somatostatin, neuropeptid Y og cholecystokinin i svins hippocampus udviser store ligheder med fordelingen hos andre pattedyr, hvorimod fordelingen af enkephalin og substans P hos svin afviger klart fra andre pattedyr, idet mosfibersystemet hos svin indeholder substans P, men ikke enkephalin, i modsætning til alle andre pattedyr, hvis mosfibersystem indeholder enkephalin, men ikke substans P. Endelig svarer fordelingen af parvalbumin hos svin til fordelingen hos andre pattedyr, mens fordelingen af calbindin-D 28k hos svin afviger fra andre pattedyr, da granulacellerne, mosfibersystemet og pyramidecellerne indeholder calbindin-D 28k hos alle andre pattedyr end svin.

I betragtning af den centrale placering af area dentata i forståelsen af patogenesen ved temporallaps epilepsi og hypoxisk-iskæmisk neurondød, er det nærliggende at foreslå anvendelse af svin med deres forholdsvis store og primatlignende area dentata som alternativ til primater i eksperimentelle undersøgelser af disse lidelser.

7. REFERENCES

Amaral D.G.: A Golgi study of cell types in the hilar region of the hippocampus in the rat. J. Comp. Neurol. 182: 851-914, 1978.

Amaral D.G. and Campbell M.J.: Transmitter systems in the primate dentate gyrus. Human Neurobiol. 5: 169-180, 1986.

Amaral D.G., Insausti R. and Cowan W.M.: The entorhinal cortex of the monkey: I. Cytoarchitectonic organization. J. Comp Neurol. 264: 326-355, 1987.

Amaral D.G., Insausti R. and Campbell M.J.: Distribution of somatostatin immunoreactivity in the human dentate gyrus. J. Neurosci. 8: 3306-3316, 1988.

Aniksztejn L., Charton G. and Ben-Ari Y.: Selective release of endogenous zinc from the hippocampal mossy fibers in situ. Brain Res. 404: 58-64, 1987.

Arai H., Emson P.C., Mountjoy C.Q., Carasso L.H. and Heizmann C.W.: Loss of parvalbumin-immunoreactive neurones from cortex in Alzheimer-type dementia. Brain Res. 418: 164-169, 1987.

Armstrong D.M., Benzing W.C., Evans J., Terry R.D., Shields D. and Hansen L.A.: Substance P and somatostatin coexist within neuritic plaques: Implications for the pathogenesis of Alzheimer's disease. Neuroscience 31: 663-671, 1989.

Arnold S.E., Hyman B.T., Flory J, Damasio A.R. and Van Hoesen G.W.: The topographical and neuroanatomical distribution of neurofibrillary tangles and neuritic plaques in the cerebral cortex of patients with Alzheimer's disease. Cerebral Cortex 1: 103-116, 1991.

Assaf S.Y. and Chung S.-H.: Release of endogenous Zn^{2+} from brain tissue during activity. Nature 308: 734-736, 1984.

Babb T.L., Brown W.J., Pretorius J., Davenport C., Lieb J.P. and Crandall P.H.: Temporal lobe volumetric cell densities in temporal lobe epilepsy. Epilepsia 25: 729-740, 1984.

Babb T.L., Pretorius J.K., Kupfer W.R. and Crandall P.H.: Glutamate decarboxylase-immunoreactive neurons are preserved in human epileptic hippocampus. J. Neurosci. 9: 2562-2574, 1989.

Baimbridge K.G. and Miller J.J.: Immunohistochemical localization of calcium-binding protein in the cerebellum, hippocampal formation and olfactory bulb of the rat. Brain Res. 245: 223-229, 1982.

Baimbridge K.G., Mody I. and Miller J.J.: Reduction of rat hippocampal calcium-binding protein following commissural, amygdala, septal, perforant path, and olfactory bulb kindling. Epilepsia 26: 460-465, 1985.

Bakst I., Morrison J.H. and Amaral D.G.: The distribution of somatostatin-like immunoreactivity in the monkey hippocampal formation. J. Comp. Neurol. 236: 423-442, 1985.

Berchtold M.W., Celio M.R. and Heizmann C.W.: Parvalbumin in human brain. J. Neurochem. 45: 235-239, 1985.

Blackstad T.W.: Commissural connections of the hippocampal region in the rat, with special reference to their mode of termination. J. Comp. Neurol. 105: 417-537, 1956.

Bogerts B., Meertz E. and Schönfeldt-Bausch R.: Basal ganglia and limbic system pathology in schizophrenia. Arch. Gen. Psychiatry 42: 784-791, 1985.

Bouras C., Vallet P.G., Hof P.R., Charnay Y., Golaz J. and Constantinidis J.: Substance P immunoreactivity in Alzheimer disease: A study in cases presenting symmetric or asymmetric cortical atrophy. Alzheimer Dis. Assoc. Disorders 4: 24-34, 1990.

Braak E., Strotkamp B. and Braak H.: Parvalbumin-immunoreactive structures in the hippocampus of the human adult. Cell Tissue Res. 264: 33-48, 1991.

Bramham C.R., Torp R., Zhang N., Storm-Mathisen J. and Ottersen O.P.: Distribution of glutamate-like immunoreactivity in excitatory hippocampal pathways: A semiquantitative electron microscopic study in rats. Neuroscience 39: 405-417, 1990.

Breazile J.E.: The cytoarchitecture of the brain stem of the domestic pig. J. Comp. Neurol. 129: 169-188, 1967.

Cassell M.D. and Brown M.W.: The distribution of Timm's stain in the nonsulphide-perfused human hippocampal formation. J. Comp. Neurol. 222: 461-471, 1984.

Cavazos J.E., Golarai G. and Sutula T.P.: Mossy fiber synaptic reorganization induced by kindling: Time course of development, progression, and permanence. J. Neurosci. 11: 2795-2803, 1991.

Chafetz M.D.: Timm's method modified for human tissue and compatible with adjacent section histofluorescence in the rat. Brain Res. Bull. 16: 19-24, 1986.

Chan-Palay V.: Somatostatin immunoreactive neurons in the human hippocampus and cortex shown by immunogold/silver intensification on vibratome sections: Coexistence with neuropeptide Y neurons, and effects in Alzheimer-type dementia. J. Comp. Neurol. 260: 201-223, 1987.

Chan-Palay V., Köhler C., Haesler U., Lang W. and Yasargil G.: Distribution of neurons and axons immunoreactive with antisera against neuropeptide Y in the normal human hippocampus. J. Comp. Neurol. 248: 360-375, 1986a.

Chan-Palay V., Lang W., Haesler U., Köhler C. and Yasargil G.: Distribution of altered hippocampal neurons and axons immunoreactive with antisera against neuropeptide Y in Alzheimer's-type dementia. J. Comp. Neurol 248: 376-394, 1986b.

Charton G., Rovira C., Ben-Ari Y. and Leviel V.: Spontaneous and evoked release of endogenous Zn^{2+} in the hippocampal mossy fiber zone of the rat in situ. Exp. Brain Res. 58: 202-205, 1985.

Christine C.W. and Choi D.W.: Effect of zinc on NMDA receptor-mediated channel currents in cortical neurons. J. Neurosci. 10: 108-116, 1990.

Coggeshall R.E.: A consideration of neural counting methods. TINS 15: 9-13, 1992.

Coleman P.D., Flood D.G. and West M.J.: Volumes of the components of the hippocampus in the aging F344 rat. J. Comp. Neurol. 266: 300-306, 1987.

Cotman C.W., Monaghan D.T., Ottersen O.P. and Storm-Mathisen J.: Anatomical organization of excitatory amino acid receptors and their pathways. TINS 10: 273-280, 1987.

Crawford I.L.: Zinc and the hippocampus: Histology, neurochemistry, pharmacology, and putative functional relevance. In: Neurobiology of the trace elements (I.E. Dreosti and R.M. Smith, eds.), Humana Press, Clifton, N.J., pp. 163-211, 1983.

Crawford I.L. and Connor J.D.: Localization and release of glutamic acid in relation to the hippocampal mossy fibre pathway. Nature 244: 442-443, 1973.

Crutcher K.A. and Davis J.N.: Target regulation of sympathetic sprouting in the rat hippocampal formation. Exp. Neurol. 75: 347-359, 1982.

Dam A.M.: Hippocampal neuron loss in epilepsy and after experimental seizures. Acta Neurol. Scand. 66: 601-642, 1982.

Damasio A.R., Eslinger P.J., Damasio H., Van Hoesen G.W. and Cornell S.: Multimodal amnesic syndrome following bilateral temporal and basal forebrain damage. Arch Neurol. 42: 252-259, 1985.

Danscher G.: Histochemical demonstration of heavy metals. A revised version of the sulphide-silver method suitable for both light and electronmicroscopy. Histochemistry 71: 1-16, 1981.

Danscher G. and Zimmer J.: An improved Timm sulphide silver method for light and electron microscopic localization of heavy metals in biological tissues. Histochemistry 55: 27-40, 1978.

deLanerolle N.C., Kim J.H., Robbins R.J. and Spencer D.D.: Hippocampal interneuron loss and plasticity in human temporal lobe epilepsy. Brain Res. 495: 387-395, 1989.

Del Fiacco M., Levanti M.C., Dessi M.L. and Zucca G.: The human hippocampal formation and parahippocampal gyrus: Localization of substance P-like immunoreactivity in newborn and adult post-mortem tissue. Neuroscience 21: 141-150, 1987.

Dilberović F., Šećerov D and Tomić V: Morphological characteristics of the gyrus dentatus in some animal species and in man. Anat. Anz. Jena 161: 231-238, 1986.

Dodds W.J.: The pig model for biomedical research. Federation Proceedings 41: 247-256, 1982.

Douglas W.R.: Of pigs and men and research: A review of applications and analogies of the pig, sus scrofa, in human medical research. Space Life Sci. 3: 226-234, 1972.

Eichenbaum H., Otto T. and Cohen N.J.: The hippocampus - what does it do? Behav. Neural Biol. 57: 2-36, 1992.

Falkai P. and Bogerts B.: Cell loss in the hippocampus of schizophrenics. Arch. Psychiatr. Neurol. Sci. 236: 154-161, 1986.

Ferrer I., Zujar M.J., Admella C. and Alcantara S.: Parvalbumin and calbindin immunoreactivity in the cerebral cortex of the hedgehog (*Erinaceus europaeus*). J. Anat. 180: 165-174, 1992.

Fitzpatrick D. and Johnson R.P.: Enkephalin-like immunoreactivity in the mossy fiber pathway of the hippocampal formation of the tree shrew (*Tupaia glis*). Neuroscience 6: 2485-2494, 1981.

Forsythe I.D., Westbrook G.L. and Mayer M.L.: Modulation of excitatory synaptic transmission by glycine and zinc in cultures of mouse hippocampal neurons. J. Neurosci. 8: 3733-3741, 1988.

Fredens K., Stengaard-Pedersen K. and Larsson L.-I.: Localization of enkephalin and cholecystokinin immunoreactivities in the perforant path terminal fields of the rat hippocampal formation. Brain Res. 304: 255-263, 1984.

Fredens K., Stengaard-Pedersen K. and Wallace M.N.: Localization of cholecystokinin in the dentate commissural-associational system of the mouse and rat. Brain Res. 401: 68-78, 1987.

Freeman T.B., Wojak J.C., Brandeis L., Michel J.P. Pearson J. and Flamm E.S.: Cross-species intracerebral grafting of embryonic swine dopaminergic neurons. Prog. Brain Res. 78: 473-477, 1988.

Freund T.F., Buzsáki G., Leon A., Baimbridge K.G. and Somogyi P.: Relationship of neuronal vulnerability and calcium binding protein immunoreactivity in ischemia. Exp. Brain Res. 83: 55-66, 1990.

Friedman B. and Price J.L.: Fiber systems in the olfactory bulb and cortex: A study in adult and developing rats, using the Timm method with the light and electron microscope. J. Comp. Neurol. 223: 88-109, 1984.

Frotscher M. and Zimmer J.: Lesion-induced mossy fibers to the molecular layer of the rat fascia dentata: Identification of postsynaptic granule cells by the Golgi-EM technique. J. Comp. Neurol. 215: 299-311, 1983.

Frotscher M., Léránth Cs., Lübbers K. and Oertel W.H.: Commissural afferents innervate glutamate decarboxylase immunoreactive non-pyramidal neurons in the guinea pig hippocampus. Neurosci. Lett. 46: 137-143, 1984.

Gall C.: The distribution of cholecystokinin-like immunoreactivity in the hippocampal formation of the guinea pig: Localization in the mossy fibers. Brain Res. 306: 73-83, 1984.

Gall C.: Seizures induce dramatic and distinctly different changes in enkephalin, dynorphin, and CCK immunoreactivities in mouse hippocampal mossy fibers. J. Neurosci. 8: 1852-1862, 1988.

Gall C.: Comparative anatomy of the hippocampus: With special reference to differences in the distributions of neuroactive peptides. In: Cerebral cortex, Vol. 8B: Comparative structure and evolution of cerebral cortex, Part II (E.G. Jones and A. Peters, eds.), Plenum Press, New York, pp. 167-213, 1990.

Gall C. and Selawski L.: Supramammillary afferents to guinea pig hippocampus contain substance P-like immunoreactivity. Neurosci. Lett. 51: 171-176, 1984.

Gall C., Brecha N., Karten H.J. and Chang K.-J.: Localization of enkephalin-like immunoreactivity to identified axonal and neuronal populations of the rat hippocampus. J. Comp. Neurol. 198: 335-350, 1981.

Gall C., Berry L.M. and Hodgson L.A.: Cholecystokinin in the mouse hippocampus: Localization in the mossy fiber and dentate commissural systems. Exp. Brain Res. 62: 431-437, 1986.

Gamrani H., Onteniente B, Seguela P., Geffard M. and Calas A.: Gamma aminobutyric acid-immunoreactivity in the rat hippocampus. A light and electron microscopic study with anti-GABA antibodies. Brain Res. 364: 30-38, 1986.

Geneser F.A.: Distribution of acetylcholinesterase in the hippocampal region of the rabbit. II. Subiculum and hippocampus. J. Comp. Neurol. 262: 90-104, 1987a.

Geneser F.A.: Distribution o f acetylcholinesterase in the hippocampal region of the rabbit. III. The dentate area. J. Comp. Neurol. 262: 594-606, 1987b.

Geneser F.A.: Histochemical distribution of zinc in the hippocampal region of the rabbit. Eur. J. Neurosci. Suppl. 6: 64, 1993.

Geneser-Jensen F.A., Haug F.-M.Š. and Danscher G.: Distribution of heavy metals in the hippocampal region of the guinea pig. A light microscope study with Timm's sulphide silver method. Z. Zellforsch. 147: 441-478, 1974.

Geneser F.A., Holm I.E. and Slomianka L.: Application of the Timm and selenium methods to the central nervous system. Neurosci. Prot. 93-050-5-01-14.

Golarai G., Cavazos J.E. and Sutula T.P.: Activation of the dentate gyrus by pentylenetetrazol evoked seizures induces mossy fiber synaptic reorganization. Brain Res. 593: 257-264, 1992.

Graham D.I.: Hypoxia and vascular disorders. In: Greenfield's Neuropathology. - Fifth Edition, (J.H. Adams and L.W. Duchen, eds.). Edward Arnold, London, pp. 153-268, 1992.

Gulyás A.I., Tóth K., Dános P. and Freund T.F.: Subpopulations of GABAergic neurons containing parvalbumin, calbindin D28k, and cholecystokinin in the rat hippocampus. J. Comp. Neurol. 312: 371-378, 1991.

Gundersen H.J.G.: Stereology of arbitrary particles. J. Microsc. 143: 3-45, 1986.

Gundersen H.J.G., Bendtsen T.F., Korbo L., Marcussen N., Møller A., Nielsen K., Nyengaard J.R., Pakkenberg B., Sørensen F.B., Vesterby A. and West M.J.:

Some new, simple and efficient stereological methods and their use in pathological research and diagnosis. APMIS 96: 379-394, 1988.

Gaarskjaer F.B., Danscher G. and West M.J.: Hippocampal mossy fibers in the regio superior of the European hedgehog. Brain Res. 237: 79-90, 1982.

Haglund L., Swanson L.W. and Köhler C.: The projection of the supramammillary nucleus to the hippocampal formation: An immunohistochemical and anterograde transport study with the lectin PHA-L in the rat. J. Comp. Neurol. 229: 171-185, 1984.

Haug F.-M.Š.: Electron microscopical localization of the zinc in hippocampal mossy fibre synapses by a modified sulfide silver procedure. Histochemie 8: 355-368, 1967.

Haug F.-M.Š.: Heavy metals in the brain. A light microscope study of the rat with Timm's sulphide silver method. Methodological considerations and cytological and regional staining patterns. Adv. Anat. Embryol. Cell Biol. 47: 1-71, 1973.

Haug F.-M.Š.: Light microscopical mapping of the hippocampal region, the pyriform cortex and the corticomedial amygdaloid nuclei of the rat with Timm's sulphide method. I. Area dentata, hippocampus and subiculum. Z. Anat. Entwickl.-Gesch. 145: 1-27, 1974.

Haug F.-M.Š.: On the normal histochemisty of trace metals in the brain. J. Hirnforsch. 16: 151-162, 1975.

Haug F.-M.Š.: Sulphide silver pattern and cytoarchitectonics of parahippocampal areas in the rat. Adv. Anat. Embryol. Cell Biol. 52: 1-73, 1976.

Haug F.-M.Š.: Sulfide silver stainable (Timm stainable) fiber systems in the brain. In: The neurobiology of zinc. Part A: Physiochemistry, anatomy and techniques (C.J. Frederickson, G.A. Howell and E. Kasarskis, eds.), Alan R. Liss, Inc., New York, pp. 213-228, 1984.

Heizmann C.W.: Parvalbumin, an intracellular calcium-binding protein; distribution, properties and possible roles in mammalian cells. Experientia 40: 910-921, 1984.

Heizmann C.W. and Braun K.: Changes in Ca^{2+}-binding proteins in human neurodegenerative disorders. TINS 15: 259-264, 1992.

Heizmann C.W and Celio M.R.: Immunolocalization of parvalbumin. Methods Enzymol. 139: 552-570, 1987.

Hereć S.: Structure of the olfactory tubercle and nucleus of the diagonal tract of Broca in the pig. Folia Morph. 26: 452-458, 1967.

Hjorth-Simonsen A.: Projection of the lateral part of the entorhinal area to the hippocampus and fascia dentata. J. Comp. Neurol. 146: 219-232, 1972.

Hjorth-Simonsen A.: Distribution of commissural afferents to the hippocampus of the rabbit. J. Comp. Neurol. 176: 495-514, 1977.

Hjorth-Simonsen A. and Jeune B.: Origin and termination of the hippocampal perforant path in the rat studied by silver impregnation. J. Comp. Neurol. 144: 215-232, 1972.

Hjorth-Simonsen A. and Laurberg S.: Commissural connection of the dentate area in the rat. J. Comp. Neurol. 174: 591-606, 1977.

Hong J.S., Yoshikawa K., Kanamatsu T., McGinty J.F., Mitchell C.L. and Sabol S.L.: Repeated electroconvulsive shocks alter the biosynthesis of enkephalin and concentration of dynorphin in the rat brain. Neuropeptides 5: 557-560, 1985.

Houser C.R., Miyashiro J.E., Swartz B.E., Walsh G.O., Rich J.R. and Delgado-Escueta A.V.: Altered patterns of dynorphin immunoreactivity suggest mossy fiber reorganization in human hippocampal epilepsy. J. Neurosci. 10: 267-282, 1990.

Howell G.A. and Frederickson C.J.: A retrograde transport method for mapping zinc-containing fiber systems in the brain. Brain Res. 515: 277-286, 1990.

Howell G.A., Welch M.G. and Frederickson C.J.: Stimulation-induced uptake and release of zinc in hippocampal slices. Nature 308: 736-738, 1984.

Huffaker T.K., Boss B.D., Morgan A.S., Neff N.T., Strecker R.E., Spence M.S.

and Miao R.: Xenografting of fetal pig ventral mesencephalon corrects motor asymmetry in the rat model of Parkinson's disease. Exp Brain Res. 77: 329-336, 1989.

Hyman B.T., Van Hoesen G.W., Damasio A.R. and Barnes C.L.: Alzheimer's disease: Cell-specific pathology isolates the hippocampal formation. Science 225: 1168-1170, 1984.

Hyman B.T., Van Hoesen G.W. and Damasio A.R.: Memory-related neural systems in Alzheimer's disease: An anatomic study. Neurology 40: 1721-1730, 1990.

Ibata Y. and Otsuka N.: Electron microscopic demonstration of zinc in the hippocampal formation using Timm's sulfide silver technique. J. Histochem. Cytochem. 17: 171-175, 1969.

Ichimiya Y., Emson P.C., Mountjoy C.Q., Lawson D.E.M. and Heizmann C.W.: Loss of calbindin-28k immunoreactive neurones from the cortex in Alzheimer-type dementia. Brain Res. 475: 156-159, 1988.

Ino T., Itoh K., Sugimoto T., Kaneko T., Kamiya H. and Mizuno N.: The supramammillary region of the cat sends substance P-like immunoreactive axons to the hippocampal formation and the entorhinal cortex. Neurosci. Lett. 90: 259-264, 1988.

Iritani S., Fujii M. and Satoh K.: The distribution of substance P in the cerebral cortex and hippocampal formation: An immunohistochemical study in the monkey and rat. Brain Res. Bull. 22: 295-303, 1989.

Jaarsma D. and Korf J.: A novel non-perfusion Timm method for human brain tissue. J. Neurosci. Meth. 35: 125-131, 1990.

Jakob H. and Beckmann H.: Prenatal developmental disturbances in the limbic allocortex in schizophrenics. J. Neural Transmission 65: 303-326, 1986.

Jande S.S., Maler L. and Lawson D.E.M.: Immunohistochemical mapping of vitamin D-dependent calcium-binding protein in brain. Nature 294: 765-767, 1981.

Johansen F.F. and Diemer N.H.: Enhancement of GABA neurotransmission after cerebral ischemia in the rat reduces loss of hippocampal CA1 pyramidal cells. Acta Neurol. Scand 84: 1-6, 1991.

Johansen F.F. and O'Hare, M.M.T.: Loss of somatal neuropeptide Y immunoreactivity in the rat hippocampus following transient cerebral ischemia. J. Neurosurg. Anesth. 1 339-345, 1989.

Johansen F.F., Zimmer J. and Diemer N.H.: Early loss of somatostatin neurons in dentate hilus after cerebral ischemia in the rat precedes CA-1 pyramidal cell loss. Acta Neuropathol. (Berl.) 73: 110-114, 1987.

Johansen F.F., Tønder N., Zimmer J., Baimbridge K.G. and Diemer N.H.: Short-term changes of parvalbumin and calbindin immunoreactivity in the rat hippocampus following cerebral ischemia. Neurosci. Lett. 120: 171-174, 1990.

Johansen F.F., Christensen T., Jensen M.S., Valente E., Jensen C.V., Nathan T., Lambert J.D.C. and Diemer N.H.: Inhibition in postischemic rat hippocampus: GABA receptors, GABA release, and inhibitory postsynaptic potentials. Exp. Brain Res. 84: 529-537, 1991.

Kanamatsu T., McGinty J.F., Mitchell C.L. and Hong J.S.: Dynorphin- and enkephalin-like immunoreactivity is altered in limbic-basal ganglia regions of rat brain after repeated electroconvulsive shock. J. Neurosci. 6: 644-649, 1986a.

Kanamatsu T., Obie J., Grimes L., McGinty J.F., Yoshikawa K., Sabol S. and Hong J.S.: Kainic acid alters the metabolism of Met[5]-enkephalin and the level of dynorphin A in the rat hippocampus. J. Neurosci. 6: 3094-3102, 1986b.

Kamphuis W., Huisman E., Wadman W.J., Heizmann C.W. and Lopes da Silva F.H.: Kindling induced changes in parvalbumin immunoreactivity in rat hippocampus and its relation to long-term decrease in GABA-immunoreactivity. Brain Res. 479: 23-34, 1989.

Kar S., Bretherton-Watt D., Gibson S.J., Steel J.H., Gentleman S.M., Roberts G.W., Valentino K., Tatemoto K., Ghatei M.A., Bloom S.R. and Polak J.M.: Novel peptide pancreastatin: Its occurrence and codistribution with chromogranin A in the central nervous system of the pig. J. Comp. Neurol. 288: 627-639, 1989.

Katsumaru H., Kosaka T., Heizmann C.W. and Hama K.: Immunocytochemical study of GABAergic neurons containing the calcium-binding protein parvalbumin in the rat hippocampus. Exp. Brain Res. 72: 347-362, 1988.

Katzman R.: Alzheimer's disease. New Engl. J. Med. 314: 964-973, 1986.

Kesslak J.P., Frederickson C.J. and Gage F.H.: Quantification of hippocampal noradrenaline and zinc changes after selective cell destruction. Exp. Brain Res. 67: 77-84, 1987.

Koh, J.-Y. and Choi D.W.: Zinc alters excitatory amino acid neurotoxicity on cortical neurons. J. Neurosci. 8: 2164-2171, 1988.

Kosaka T., Hama, K. and Wu J.-Y.: GABAergic synaptic boutons in the granule cell layer of rat dentate gyrus. Brain Res. 293: 353-359, 1984.

Kosaka T., Kosaka K., Tateishi K., Hamaoka Y., Yanaihara N., Wu J.-Y. and Hama K.: GABAergic neurons containing CCK-8-like and/or VIP-like immunoreactivities in the rat hippocampus and dentate gyrus. J. Comp. Neurol. 239: 420-430, 1985.

Kosaka T., Wu J.-Y. and Benoit R.: GABAergic neurons containing somatostatin-like immunorectivity in the rat hippocampus and dentate gyrus. Exp. Brain Res. 71: 388-398, 1988.

Kosaka T., Katsumaru H., Hama K., Wu J.-Y. and Heizmann C.W.: GABAergic neurons containing the Ca^{2+}-binding protein parvalbumin in the rat hippocampus and dentate gyrus. Brain Res. 419. 119-130, 1987.

Krettek J.E. and Price J.L.: Projections from the amygdaloid complex and adjacent olfactory structures to the entorhinal complex and to the subiculum in the rat and cat. J. Comp. Neurol. 172: 723-752, 1977.

Krieger D.T.: Brain peptides: What, where, and why? Science 222: 975-985, 1983.

Kruska D.: Vergleichende cytoarchitektonische Untersuchungen an Gehirnen von Wild- und Hausschweinen. Z. Anat. Entwickl.-Gesch. 131: 291-324, 1970.

Köhler C., Eriksson L., Davies S. and Chan-Palay V.: Neuropeptide Y innervation of the hippocampal region in the rat and monkey brain. J. Comp. Neurol. 244: 384-400, 1986.

Köhler C., Eriksson L.G., Davies S. and Chan-Palay V.: Colocalization of neuropeptide tyrosine and somatostatin immunoreactivity in neurons of individual subfields of the rat hippocampal region. Neurosci. Lett 78: 1-6, 1987.

Larsson, L.-I.: Peptide immunocytochemistry, Vol. 13, Progress in histochemistry and cytochemistry. Gustav Fischer Verlag, Stuttgart, 1981.

Laurberg S. and Sørensen K.E.: Associational and commissural collaterals of neurons in the hippocampal formation (hilus fasciae dentatae and subfield CA3). Brain Res. 212: 287-300, 1981.

Laurberg S. and Zimmer J.: Aberrant hippocampal mossy fibers in cats. Brain Res. 188: 555-559, 1980.

Leranth C. and Ribak C.E.: Calcium-binding proteins are concentrated in the CA2 field of the monkey hippocampus: a possible key to this region's resistance to epileptic damage. Exp. Brain Res. 85: 129-136, 1991.

Lorente de Nó, R.: Studies on the structure of the cerebral cortex. I. The area entorhinalis. J. Psychol. Neurol. (Lpz.) 45: 381-438, 1933.

Lorente de Nó, R.: Studies on the structure of the cerebral cortex. II. Continuation of the study of the ammonic system. J. Psychol. Neurol. (Lpz.) 46: 113-177, 1934.

Lothman E.W., Bertram E.H., III and Stringer J.L.: Functional anatomy of hippocampal seizures. Prog. Neurobiol. 37: 1-82, 1991.

Lotstra F. and Vanderhaeghen J.-J.: Distribution of immunoreactive cholecystokinin in the human hippocampus. Peptides 8: 911-920, 1987.

Lotstra F., Mailleux P. and Vanderhaeghen J.-J.: Substance P neurons in the human hippocampus: An immunohistochemical analysis in the infant and adult. J. Chem. Neuroanat. 1: 111-123, 1988.

Lotstra F., Schiffmann S.N. and Vanderhaeghen J.-J.: Neuropeptide Y containing neurons in the human infant hippocampus. Brain Res. 478: 211-226, 1989.

Marksteiner J., Ortler M., Bellmann R. and Sperk G.: Neuropeptide Y biosynthesis is markedly induced in mossy fibers during temporal lobe epilepsy of the rat. Neurosci. Lett. 112: 143-148, 1990.

Mayhew T.M.: A review of recent advances in stereology for quantifying neural structure. J. Neurocytol. 21: 313-328, 1992.

McGinty J.F., Henriksen S.J., Goldstein A., Terenius L. and Bloom F.E.: Dynorphin is contained within hippocampal mossy fibers: Immunochemical alterations after kainic acid administration and colchicine-induced neurotoxicity. Proc. Natl. Acad. Sci. U.S.A. 80: 589-593, 1983.

McGinty J.F., Henriksen S.J. and Chavkin C.: Is there an interaction between zinc and opioid peptides in hippocampal neurons? In: The neurobiology of zinc. Part A: Physiochemistry, anatomy, and techniques (C.J. Frederickson, G.A. Howell and E.J. Kasarskis, eds.), Alan R. Liss, Inc., New York, pp. 73-89, 1984.

McLean S, Rothman R.B., Jacobson A.E., Rice K.C. and Herkenham M.: Distribution of opiate receptor subtypes and enkephalin and dynorphin immunoreactivity in the hippocampus of squirrel, guinea pig, rat, and hamster. J. Comp. Neurol. 255: 497-510, 1987.

Meldrum B.S. and Bruton C.J.: Epilepsy. In: Greenfield's Neuropathology. Fifth Edition, (J.H. Adams and L.W. Duchen, eds.). Edward Arnold, London, pp. 1246-1283, 1992.

Miller J.J. and Baimbridge K.G.: Biochemical and immunohistochemical correlates of kindling-induced epilepsy: role of calcium binding protein. Brain Res. 278: 322-326, 1983.

Milner B.: Memory and the medial temporal regions of the brain. In: Biology of memory (K.H. Pribram and D.E. Broadbent, eds.), Academic Press, New York, pp. 29-50, 1970.

Mizusawa H., Hirano A. and Llena J.F.: Involvement of hippocampus in Creutzfeldt-Jakob disease. J. Neurol. Sci. 82: 13-26, 1987.

Nitsch R., Soriano E. and Frotscher M.: The parvalbumin-containing nonpyramidal neurons in the rat hippocampus. Anat. Embryol. 181: 413-425, 1990.

Niwa M., Shigematsu K., Kurihara M., Kataoka Y., Maeda T., Nakao,K., Imura H., Matsuo H., Tsuchiyama H. and Ozaki M.: Receptor autoradiographic evidence of specific brain natriuretic peptide binding sites in the porcine subfornical organ. Neurosci. Lett. 95: 113-118, 1988.

Olney J.W.: Excitotoxins: An overview. In: Excitotoxins (K. Fuxe, P. Roberts and R. Schwarcz, eds.), Macmillan Press, London, pp. 82-96, 1983.

Orzi F., Zoli M., Passarelli F., Ferraguti F., Fieschi C. and Agnati L.F.: Repeated electroconvulsive shock increases glial fibrillary acidic protein, ornithine decarboxylase, somatostatin and cholecystokinin immunoreactivities in the hippocampal formation of the rat. Brain Res. 533: 223-231, 1990.

Palacios J.M. and Mengod G.: Radiohistochemistry of receptors in the hippocampus: Focus on the cholinergic receptors. In: The hippocampus - New vistas (V. Chan-Palay and C. Köhler, eds.), Alan R. Liss, Inc., New York, pp. 207-224, 1989.

Palmieri G., Farina V., Panu R., Asole A., Sanna L., de Riu P.L. and Gabbi C.: Course and termination of the pyramidal tract in the pig. Arch. Anat. Microsc. 75: 167-176, 1987.

Pérez-Clausell J. and Danscher G.: Intravesicular localization of zinc in rat telencephalic boutons. A histochemical study. Brain Res 337: 91-98, 1985.

Pérez-Clausell J. and Danscher G.: Release of zinc sulphide accumulations into synaptic clefts after in vivo injection of sodium sulphide. Brain Res. 362: 358-361, 1986.

Peters S., Koh J. and Choi D.W.: Zinc selectively blocks the action of N-methyl-D-aspartate on cortical neurons. Science 236: 589-593, 1987.

Pickel V.M.: Immunocytochemical methods. In: Neuroanatomical tract-tracing methods (L. Heimer and M.J. Robards, eds.), Plenum Press, New York and London, pp. 483-509, 1981.

Pitkänen A. and Amaral D.G.: Distribution of parvalbumin-immunoreactive cells and fibers in the monkey temporal lobe: The hippocampal formation. J. Comp. Neurol. 331: 37-74, 1993.

Price D.L., Martin L.J., Sisodia S.S., Wagster M.V., Koo E.H., Walker L.C., Koliatsos V. and Cork L.C.: Aged non-human primates: An animal model of age-associated neurodegenerative disease. Brain Pathol. 1: 287-296, 1991.

Quigley B.J., Jr. and Kowall N.W.: Substance P-like immunoreactive neurons are depleted in Alzheimer's disease cerebral cortex. Neuroscience 41: 41-60, 1991.

Rami A., Bréhier A., Thomasset M. and Rabié A.: The comparative immunocytochemical distribution of 28 kDa cholecalcin (CaBP) in the hippocampus of rat, guinea pig and hedgehog. Brain Res. 422: 149-153, 1987.

Ramón y Cajal S.: Estructura del asta de Ammon. Anal. Soc. Esp. Hist. Nat. Madr. 22: 53-114, 1893.

Ramón y Cajal S.: The structure of Ammon's horn. (English translation of Ramón y Cajal, 1893), Charles C. Thomas, Springfield, Il., 1968.

Ribak C.E. and Peterson G.M.: Intragranular mossy fibers in rats and gerbils form synapses with the somata and proximal dendrites of basket cells in the dentate gyrus. Hippocampus 1: 355-364, 1991.

Ribak C.E. and Seress L.: Five types of basket cell in the hippocampal dentate gyrus: A combined Golgi and electron microscopic study. J. Neurocytol. 12: 577-597, 1983.

Ribak C.E., Vaughn J.E. and Saito K.: Immunocytochemical localization of glutamic acid decarboxylase in neuronal somata following colchicine inhibition of axonal transport. Brain Res. 140: 315-332, 1978.

Ribak C.E., Nitsch R. and Seress L.: Proportion of parvalbumin-positive basket cells in the GABAergic innervation of pyramidal and granule cells of the rat hippocampal formation. J. Comp. Neurol. 300: 449-461, 1990.

Ribak C.E., Seress L. and Leranth C.: Electron microscopic immuno-cytochemical study of the distribution of parvalbumin-containing neurons and axon terminals in the primate dentate gyrus and Ammon's horn. J. Comp. Neurol. 327: 298-321, 1993.

Robbins R.J., Brines M.L., Kim J.H., Adrian T., de Lanerolle N., Welsh S. and Spencer D.D.: A selective loss of somatostatin in the hippocampus of patients with temporal lobe epilepsi. Ann. Neurol. 29: 325-332, 1991.

Rosene D.L. and van Hoesen G.W.: The hippocampal formation of the primate brain. A review of some comparative aspects of cytoarchitecture and connections. In: Cerebral cortex, Vol. 6. Further aspects of cortical function, including hippocampus (E.G. Jones and A. Peters, eds.), Plenum Press, New York, pp. 345-456, 1987.

Rungby J., Slomianka L., Danscher G., Andersen A.H. and West M.J.: A quantitative evaluation of the neurotoxic effect of silver on the volumes of the components of the developing rat hippocampus. Toxicology 43: 261-268, 1987.

Sakamoto N., Michel J.-P., Kopp N., Tohyama M. and Pearson J.: Substance P- and enkephalin-immunoreactive neurons in the hippocampus and related areas of the human infant brain. Neuroscience 22: 80-811, 1987.

Schaffer K.: Beitrag zur Histologie der Ammonshornformation. Arch. Mikrosk. Anat. 39: 611-632, 1892.

Scharfman H.E. and Schwartzkroin P.A.: Protection of dentate hilar cells from prolonged stimulation by intracellular calcium chelation. Science 246: 257-260, 1989.

Schlander M. and Frotscher M.: Non-pyramidal neurons in the guinea pig hippocampus. A combined Golgi-electron microscope study. Anat. Embryol. 174: 35-47, 1986.

Schmechel D.E., Vickrey B.G., Fitzpatrick D. and Elde R.P.: GABAergic neurons of mammalian cerebral cortex: Widespread subclass defined by somatostatin content. Neurosci. Lett. 47: 227-232, 1984.

Schmidt-Kastner R. and Freund T.F.: Selective vulnerability of the hippocampus in brain ischemia. Neuroscience 40: 599-636, 1991.

Schurr A. and Rigor B.M.: The mechanism of cerebral hypoxic-ischemic damage. Hippocampus 2: 221-228, 1992.

Scoville W.B. and Milner B.: Loss of recent memory after bilateral hippocampal lesions. J. Neurol. Neurosurg. psychiat. 20: 11-21, 1957.

Seeger J.: Zytoarchitektur und Topographie ausgewählter Kerngebiete des ventromedialen Hypothalamus des Schweines (Sus scrofa domestica). J. Hirnforsch. 31: 601-611, 1990.

Seress L., Gulyás A.I. and Freund T.F.: Parvalbumin- and calbindin D_{28k}-immunoreactive neurons in the hippocampal formation of the Macaque monkey. J. Comp. Neurol. 313: 162-177, 1991.

Seress L., Gulyás A.I. and Freund T.F.: Pyramidal neurons are immunoreactive for calbindin D_{28k} in the CA1 subfield of the human hippocampus. Neurosci. Lett. 138: 257-260, 1992.

Shepherd G.M.: Neurobiology, Second Edition. Oxford University Press, New York, Oxford, 1988.

Siesjö B.K. and Bengtsson F.: Calcium fluxes, calcium antagonists, and calcium-related pathology in brain ischemia, hypoglycemia, and spreading depression: A unifying hypothesis. J. Cereb. Blood Flow Metab. 9: 127-140, 1989.

Slevin J.T. and Kasarskis E.J.: Effects of zinc on markers of glutamate and aspartate neurotransmission in rat hippocampus. Brain Res. 334: 281-286, 1985.

Slomianka L.: Neurons of origin of zinc-containing pathways and the distribution of zinc-containing boutons in the hippocampal region of the rat. Neuroscience 48: 325-352, 1992.

Slomianka L., Rungby J., West M.J., Danscher G. and Andersen A.H.: Dose-dependent bimodal effect of low-level lead exposure on the developing hippocampal region of the rat: A volumetric study. NeuroToxicology 10: 177-190, 1989.

Slomianka L., Danscher G. and Frederickson C.J.: Labeling of the neurons of origin of zinc-containing pathways by intraperitoneal injections of sodium selenite. Neuroscience 38: 843-854, 1990.

Slomianka L., Rungby J., Edelfors S. and Ravn-Jonsen A.: Late postnatal growth in the dentate area of the rat hippocampus compensates for volumetric changes caused by early postnatal toluene exposure. Toxicology 74: 203-208, 1992.

Sloviter R.S.: Decreased hippocampal inhibition and a selective loss of interneurons in experimental epilepsy. Science 235: 73-76, 1987.

Sloviter R.S.: Chemically defined hippocampal interneurons and their possible relationship to seizure mechanisms. In: The hippocampus - New vistas (V. Chan-Palay and C. Köhler, eds.), Alan R. Liss, Inc., New York, pp. 443-461, 1989a.

Sloviter R.S.: Calcium-binding protein (calbindin-D_{28k}) and parvalbumin immunocytochemistry: Localization in the rat hippocampus with specific reference to the selective vulnerability of hippocampal neurons to seizure activity. J. Comp. Neurol. 280: 183-196, 1989b.

Sloviter R.S.: Permanently altered hippocampal structure, excitability, and inhibition after experimental status epilepticus in the rat: The "dormant basket cell" hypothesis and its possible relevance to temporal lobe epilepsy. Hippocampus 1: 41-66, 1991.

Sloviter R.S. and Nilaver G.: Immunocytochemical localization of GABA-, cholecystokinin-, vasoactive intestinal polypeptide-, and somatostatin-like immunoreactivity in the area dentata and hippocampus of the rat. J. Comp. Neurol. 256: 42-60, 1987.

Sloviter R.S., Sollas A.L., Barbaro N.M. and Laxer K.D.: Calcium-binding protein (calbindin-D28K) and parvalbumin immunocytochemistry in the normal and epileptic human hippocampus. J. Comp. Neurol. 308: 381-396, 1991.

Smart T.G.: A novel modulatory binding site for zinc on the $GABA_A$ receptor complex in cultured rat neurones. J. Physiol. 447: 587-625, 1992.

Smart T.G. and Constanti A.: Differential effect of zinc on the vertebrate GABA$_A$-receptor complex. Br. J. Pharmacol 99: 643-654, 1990.

Solnitzky O.: The thalamic nuclei of *Sus scrofa*. J. Comp. Neurol. 69: 121-169, 1938.

Sommer W.: Erkrankung des Ammonshorns als aetiologisches Moment der Epilepsie. Archiv für Psychiatrie und Nervenheilkunde 10: 631-675, 1880.

Somogyi P., Smith A.D., Nunzi M.G., Gorio A., Takagi H. and Wu J.Y.: Glutamate decarboxylase immunoreactivity in the hippocampus of the cat: Distribution of immunoreactive synaptic terminals with special reference to the axon initial segment of pyramidal neurons. J. Neurosci. 3: 1450-1468, 1983.

Somogyi P., Hodgson A.J., Smith A.D., Nunzi M.G., Gorio A. and Wu J.-Y.: Different populations of GABAergic neurons in the visual cortex and hippocampus of cat contain somatostatin- or cholecystokinin-immunoreactive material. J. Neurosci. 4: 2590-2603, 1984.

Squire L.R.: Memory: neural organization and behavior. In: Handbook of physiology, Section 1, Vol. V (V.B. Mountcastle, F. Plum and S.R. Geiger, eds.), American Physiological Society, Bethesda, Maryland, pp. 295-371, 1987.

Squire L.R.: Memory and the hippocampus: A synthesis from findings with rats, monkeys, and humans: Psychol. Rev. 99: 195-231, 1992.

Squire L.R. and Zola-Morgan S.: The medial temporal lobe memory system. Science 253: 1380-1386, 1991.

Stengaard-Pedersen K., Fredens K. and Larsson L.-L.: Comparative localization of enkephalin and cholecystokinin immunoreactivities and heavy metals in the hippocampus. Brain Res. 273: 81-96, 1983.

Stephan H.: Vergleichende Untersuchungen über den Feinbau des Hirnes von Wild- und Haustieren. (Nach Studien am Schwein und Schaf.) Zool. Jb., Abt. Anat. Ontog. 71: 487-586, 1951.

Stephan H.: Evolutionary trends in limbic structures. Neurosci. Biobehav. Rev. 7: 367-374, 1983.

Stephan H. and Manolescu J.: Comparative investigations on hippocampus in insectivores and primates. Z. Mikrosk. Anat. Forsch. 94: 1025-1050, 1980.

Sternberger L.A.: Immunocytochemistry. John Wiley & Sons, New York, 1979.

Steward O.: Topographic organization of the projections from the entorhinal area to the hippocampal formation of the rat. J. Comp. Neurol. 167: 285-314, 1976.

Storm-Mathisen J. and Ottersen O.P.: Neurotransmitters in the hippocampal formation. In: Cortical integration (F. Reinoso-Suárez and C. Ajmone-Marsan, eds.), Raven Press, New York, pp. 105-130, 1984.

Storm-Mathisen J., Leknes A.K., Bore A.T., Vaaland J.L., Edminson P., Haug F.-M.Š. and Ottersen O.P.: First visualization of glutamate and GABA in neurones by immunocytochemistry. Nature 301: 517-520, 1983.

Sutula T., Xiao-Xian H., Cavazos J. and Scott G.: Synaptic reorganization in the hippocampus induced by abnormal functional activity. Science 239: 1147-1150, 1988.

Sutula T., Cascino G., Cavazos J., Parada I. and Ramirez L.: Mossy fiber synaptic reorganization in the epileptic human temporal lobe. Ann. Neurol. 26: 321-330, 1989.

Tauck D.L. and Nadler J.V.: Evidence of functional mossy fiber sprouting in hippocampal formation of kainic acid-treated rats. J. Neurosci. 5: 1016-1022, 1985.

Tielen A.M., van Leeuwen F.W. and Lopes da Silva F.H.: The localization of leucine-enkephalin immunoreactivity within the guinea pig hippocampus. Exp. Brain Res. 48: 288-295, 1982.

Timm F.: Zur Histochemie der Schwermetalle. Das Sulfid-Silber-Verfahren. Dtsch. Z. Ges. Gerichtl. Med. 46: 706-711, 1958.

Tomlinson B.E.: Ageing and the dementias. In: Greenfield's Neuropathology. - Fifth Edition, (J.H. Adams and L.W. Duchen, eds.). Edward Arnold, London, pp. 1284-1410, 1992.

Tóth K. and Freund T.F.: Calbindin D_{28k}-containing nonpyramidal cells in the rat hippocampus: Their immunoreactivity for GABA and projection to the medial septum. Neuroscience 49: 793-805, 1992.

Tumbleson M.E.: Swine in biomedical research, Vol. 1-3. Plenum Press, New York and London, 1986.

Turgeon S.M. and Albin R.L.: Zinc modulates $GABA_B$ binding in rat brain. Brain Res. 30: 30-34, 1992.

van Daal J.H.H.M., Zandering H.E.A., Jenks B.G. and van Abeelen J.H.F.: Distribution of dynorphin B and methionine-enkephalin in the mouse hippocampus: Influence of genotype. Neurosci. Lett. 97: 241-244, 1989.

van Eerdenburg F.J.C.M., Poot P., Molenaar G.J., van Leeuwen F.W. and Swaab D.F.: A vasopressin and oxytocin containing nucleus in the pig hypothalamus that shows neuronal changes during puberty. J. Comp. Neurol. 301: 138-146, 1990.

van Eerdenburg F.J.C.M., Swaab D.F. and van Leeuwen F.W.: Distribution of vasopressin and oxytocin cells and fibres in the hypothalamus of the domestic pig (*Sus scrofa*). J. Comp. Neurol. 318: 138-146, 1992.

van Groen T. and Wyss J.M.: Species differenes in hippocampal commissural connections. Studies in rat, guinea pig, rabbit, and cat. J. Comp. Neurol. 267: 322-334, 1988.

van Hoesen G.W. and Hyman B.T.: Hippocampal formation: anatomy and the patterns of pathology in Alzheimer's disease. Prog. Brain Res. 83: 445-457, 1990.

Victor M., Angevine J.B., Jr., Mancall E.L. and Fisher C.M.: Memory loss with lesions of hippocampal formation. Arch. Neurol. 5: 26-45, 1961.

Vincent S.R., Kimura H. and McGeer E.G.: Organization of substance P fibers with in the hippocampal formation demonstrated with a biotin-avidin immunoperoxidase technique. J. Comp. Neurol. 199: 113-123, 1981.

Volpe B.T. and Petito C.K.: Dementia with bilateral medial temporal lobe ischemia. Neurology 35: 1793-1797, 1985.

Wanscher B., Kragh J., Barry D.I., Bolwig T. and Zimmer J.: Increased somatostatin and enkephalin-like immunoreactivity in the rat hippocampus following hippocampal kindling. Neurosci. Lett. 118: 33-36, 1990.

Weiss J.H., Koh J.-Y., Christine C.W. and Choi D.W.: Zinc and LTP. Nature 338: 212, 1989.

West M.J.: Stereological studies of the hippocampus: a comparison of the hippocampal subdivisions of diverse species including hedgehogs, laboratory rodents, wild mice, and men. Prog. Brain Res. 83: 13-36, 1990.

West M.J.: New stereological methods for counting neurons. Neurobiol. Aging 14: 275-285, 1993a.

West M.J.: Regionally specific loss of neurons in the aging human hippocampus. Neurobiol. Aging 14: 287-293, 1993b.

West M.J. and Gundersen H.J.G.: Unbiased stereological estimation of the number of neurons in the human hippocampus. J. Comp. Neurol. 296: 1-22, 1990.

West M.J., Gaarskjaer F.B. and Danscher G.: The Timm-stained hippocampus of the European hedgehog: A basal mammalian form. J. Comp. Neurol. 226: 477-488, 1984.

West M.J., Slomianka L. and Gundersen H.J.G.: Unbiased stereological estimation of the total number of neurons in the subdivisions of the rat hippocampus using the optical fractionator. Anat. Rec. 231: 482-497, 1991.

Westbrook G.L. and Mayer M.L.: Micromolar concentrations of Zn^{2+} antagonize NMDA and GABA responses of hippocampal neurons. Nature 328: 640-643, 1987.

White J.D., Gall C.M. and McKelvy J.F.: Enkephalin biosynthesis and enkephalin gene expression are increased in hippocampal mossy fibers following a unilateral lesion of the hilus. J. Neurosci. 7: 753-759, 1987.

Witter M.P.: A survey of the anatomy of the hippocampal formation, with emphasis on the septotemporal organization of its intrinsic and extrinsic connections. In: Excitatory amino acids and epilepsy (R. Schwarcz and Y. Ben-Ari, eds.), Plenum Press, New York, pp. 67-82, 1986.

Wolf G. and Schmidt W.: Zinc and glutamate dehydrogenase in putative glutamatergic brain structures. Acta Histochem. (Jena) 72: 15-23, 1983.

Woolsey C.N. and Fairman D.: Contralateral, ipsilateral, and bilateral representation of cutaneous receptors in somatic areas I and II of the cerebral cortex of pig, sheep, and other mammals. Surgery 19: 684-702, 1946.

Yanagihara M. and Niimi K.: Substance P-like immunoreactive projection to the hippocampal formation from the posterior hypothalamus in the cat. Brain Res. Bull. 22: 689-694, 1989.

Zimmer J.: Ipsilateral afferents to the commissural zone of the fascia dentata, demonstrated in decommissurated rats by silver impregnation. J. Comp. Neurol. 142: 393-416, 1971.

Zola-Morgan S., Squire L.R. and Amaral D.G.: Human amnesia and the medial temporal region: Enduring memory impairment following a bilateral lesion limited to field CA1 of the hippocampus. J. Neurosci. 6: 2950-2967, 1986.

Østergaard K., Holm I.E. and Zimmer J.: Tyrosine hydroxylase and acetyl-cholinesterase in the domestic pig mesencephalon: An immunocytochemical and histochemical study. J. Comp. Neurol. 322: 149-166, 1992.